Essential Oils for Beginners

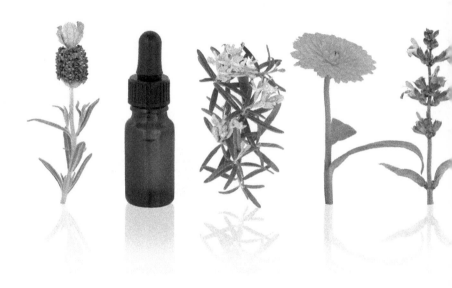

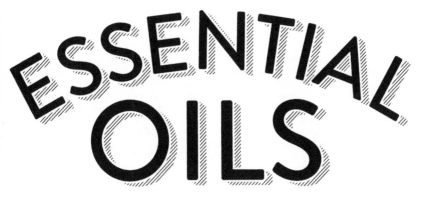

for Beginners

The Guide to Get Started with Essential Oils and Aromatherapy

ALTHEA PRESS

Contents

Oils, Recipes, and Remedies

Introduction

For thousands of years, people have been using essential oils to enhance physical, emotional, mental, and spiritual health. Only recently has science begun to discover how these volatile aromatic liquids and the precious chemical compounds they contain work to affect both body and mind.

Perhaps you are interested in using these delightfully scented oils primarily for aromatherapy, or maybe you want to learn how to create a wide variety of therapeutic products and solutions for enhancing beauty the natural way. Within these pages, you'll find a wealth of valuable information about the world's best-loved essential oils, along with more than a hundred tips for using them with confidence.

Each essential oil described in this book may be used for a variety of purposes. For example, pure peppermint essential oil is well known for its ability to soothe digestive discomfort, relieve inflammation and pain caused by arthritic conditions, and give fresh flavor to a variety of products, ranging from candy to toothpaste. This book is a comprehensive resource you can refer to whether you need a natural remedy for treating a headache or soothing cold symptoms, or even for helping minor wounds heal rapidly.

Sourced from plants, healthy for our planet, and naturally effective, essential oils are versatile and convenient. By choosing to use these fragrant gifts from nature's abundant apothecary to replace chemical-based products whenever possible, you open yourself, your family, and even companion animals up to total well-being.

CHAPTER ONE

Essential Oils and How They Work

WHAT IS AN ESSENTIAL OIL?

Essential oils are more than just highly concentrated plant extracts. Most possess potent medicinal qualities, and many are valued for their exceptional cosmetic qualities. While the whole plants or plant parts they are derived from possess beneficial qualities, essential oils are much more powerful.

Sometimes referred to as ethereal oils or volatile oils, essential oils carry the actual essence or fragrance of the plants from which they are extracted. A few popular essential oils are derived from whole plants, but most are derived from specific sections of the plants for which they are named. Some essential oils, including almond and nutmeg oils, come from seeds. Many, including patchouli, eucalyptus, and tea tree oils, are extracted from leaves. Still others come from wood, flowers, resin, or roots. Some plants, including cinnamon and bitter orange, are used as sources for more than one distinct type of essential oil.

Professional practitioners use approximately three hundred essential oils to treat a vast range of illnesses, but home practitioners typically use between ten and twenty essential oils on a regular basis. Some favorites include lavender, eucalyptus, clary sage, and orange essential oils.

A BRIEF HISTORY

Cave paintings discovered in Lascaux, France, suggest that prehistoric people used medicinal plants on a daily basis. These fascinating images have been carbon dated to approximately 18,000 BCE.

Humans have possessed an understanding of the healing power of plants for thousands of years. While it is not clear when essential oils were first distilled, we know that these oils were used in various cultures, and we know that they were used for religious ceremonies as well as for healing purposes.

Herbs and Essential Oils in Ancient Times

The Egyptian people are widely renowned for their achievements, so it might not come as a surprise that ancient Egyptians were among the first to use essential oils. In fact, records show that aromatic oils were part of daily life in Egypt as early as 4500 BCE. Cinnamon, myrrh, sandalwood, and frankincense were treasured favorites; they were of such great value that they were sometimes purchased with pure gold.

In Egypt, pure essential oils were believed to be sacred, and only high priests and royalty had the authority to use them; each deity was assigned a signature essential oil blend. Images and carvings of gods and goddesses were frequently anointed with precious oils during religious ceremonies. Each pharaoh used a variety of unique essential oil blends during meditation and intimacy, and even during preparation for war.

Around 3000 BCE, scholars in India developed the science of Ayurveda, which relies heavily on curative potions containing a wide variety of essential oils. Ancient Vedic literature lists more than seven hundred curative substances, including some of today's favorites, such as ginger and cinnamon essential oils.

In China, aromatic herbs and essential oils made their way into remedies for a whole host of ailments. Many of these compounds are still used by today's Eastern medicine practitioners. Chinese scholars first recorded the use of essential oils between 2697 and 2597 BCE, during Huang Ti's reign, and the fabled *Suwen*, or *Yellow Emperor's Classic of Internal Medicine*, remains a significant text today.

Essential oils are mentioned in both the New and Old Testaments of the Bible—over two hundred times. Some very popular biblical essential oils are cedarwood, cinnamon, fir, frankincense, myrrh, and spikenard. These oils were used for anointing, for religious purposes, and, it seems, for the pure enjoyment of their fragrances. They were also highly valued as gifts; in the story of the Magi, the precious gifts they brought to Jesus of Nazareth at his birth included frankincense and myrrh.

Greek and Roman ancients also used essential oils, mostly for aromatherapy, therapeutic massage, personal hygiene, and medicine. Essential oil of myrrh was blended into an ointment for battlefield use; it proved an effective remedy for preventing post-injury infections.

We know Hippocrates as the "Father of Medicine." Between 500 and 400 BCE, he documented the medicinal effects of essential oils and elements from over three hundred plants, many of which are still popular today. Hippocrates taught his students that "a perfumed bath and a scented massage every day is the way to good health." His wisdom continues to influence modern medicine in the form of the Hippocratic Oath taken by doctors.

Galen was an influential Greek medical practitioner. Born in 131 CE and educated in Alexandria and Smyrna, he gained fame during his tenure as the surgeon to the gladiators of Pergamos. Thanks to Galen's vast knowledge of the effective use of essential oils and other medicines, no gladiator died of infection while under his care. Galen's success led him to an assignment as personal physician to Roman Emperor Marcus Aurelius. He remained a part of the Emperor's court for the rest of his life, which he spent composing a vast body of medical texts that included plants in various medicinal categories. Though Galen died around 201 CE, his work lives on in the form of Galenic medicine, which is still practiced in India and Pakistan.

Essential Oils, Aromatherapy, and the Dawn of Modern Medicine

When Rome fell, physicians fled, carrying books by Hippocrates and Galen with them. These books made their way into Persia, where they were translated into several languages for distribution to scholars. Ali ibn Sina, who was often referred to as Avicenna the Arab, was a child prodigy born in 980 CE. He was educated as a physician and is said to have begun practicing medicine at age twelve. Ibn Sina catalogued approximately eight hundred plants, describing their effects on the human body in detail. He's also credited with refining and recording traditional distillation methods for extracting pure, high-quality essential oils from aromatic plants.

Europeans gained firsthand knowledge of essential oils and herbal medicines after crusading knights visited the Middle East. These knights and their armies began wearing and carrying perfumes, and many acquired knowledge of distillation techniques.

During the bubonic plague epidemic of the 1400s, desperate doctors decided to try Ayurvedic blends in place of ineffective medicines. These ancient remedies, which included essential oils of camphor, meadowsweet, rosemary, and lavender, proved to be effective. At the same time, frankincense and Scots pine were burned in the streets to ward off evil spirits. Fewer people died of the plague in areas where this practice was common.

Nicholas Culpeper's 1653 book *Complete Herbal* offers detailed remedies for many medical conditions. These venerable tonics contain essential oils and other effective plant-based compounds that are still widely used today.

The powerful therapeutic properties of essential oils were rediscovered in 1910, when French chemist René-Maurice Gattefossé badly burned his hands in a laboratory explosion and gangrene quickly developed. Gattefossé subsequently treated his hands with a single application of lavender oil, and healing began swiftly. Following this incident, Gattefossé and a colleague conducted further research on the healing properties of lavender essential oil before introducing it to French hospitals.

Later, Parisian doctor Jean Valnet used therapeutic-grade essential oils to treat injured soldiers during World War II. Two of Valnet's students, Dr. Paul Belaiche and Dr. Jean-Claude Lapraz, conducted extensive research, examining essential oils for their antiviral, antibacterial, antifungal, and antiseptic properties. They concluded that these powerful natural substances have substantial healing capabilities.

The using of aromatherapy and essential oils in North America is a fascinating one. We know that Native Americans relied heavily upon nature's pharmacy, utilizing plants to increase well-being in a variety of ways. Echinacea, which is used today in a variety of forms, including whole herb and essential oil, was a favorite treatment for headaches, including painful migraines. Skunk cabbage was used to treat nervous disorders, horsemint was applied to ease back pain, and wild cherry was used to treat coughs. White pine, which Native Americans used for treating colds, remains a popular aromatherapy cold treatment today. If you've ever used arnica to help bruises, you are using a well-known Native American remedy.

When European settlers came to North America, they brought favorite European herbs with them. At first, these precious plants were their only source of medicine, and the plants were also used to make food more palatable. Pennyroyal and wormwood were useful for controlling fleas and other insects. Later records show that in 1631, John Winthrop, Jr. of Suffolk ordered a vast amount of seeds to be taken to America's Massachusetts Bay Colony. Among the forty-eight plant species he ordered at a cost of £160, which was a fortune in those days, were rosemary, clary sage, angelica root, hyssop, catnip, and lovage—all of which are available as essential oils today.

As it turns out, the ancients and those who followed the pathways they laid were right. Many bacteria, fungi, and viruses die when placed in contact with certain essential oils, particularly when those oils contain terpenes, thymol, carvacrol, and phenols. Essential oils and chemical reproductions of their active ingredients are widely used in compounding modern pharmaceuticals. Extensive studies and clinical investigations are ongoing, and thanks to modern technology, many of today's medical professionals incorporate remedies containing essential oils into holistic practice.

THE POWER OF ESSENTIAL OILS

Every essential oil contains approximately one hundred different components, each of which acts on the body in different ways. Aromatic chemicals derived from phenylpropane are the precursors of the amino acids that connect with one another to form nearly all the body's structures.

Complex Natural Substances

On a chemical level, our bodies and essential oils are made from many of the same substances, including complex chemicals called terpineols, which are naturally occurring alcohols that play a vital role in the body's production of vitamins, energy, and hormones. They are produced during the constant process of cellular respiration, and they contribute to the body's cellular energy supply, aiding in processes such as metabolism and healing. These important chemicals are also found in many essential oils, as plants produce them during growth. They are very easy for the human body to absorb and use for both nourishment and healing.

Despite their complexity, these oils are for the most part noninvasive and nontoxic, though there are a select few derived from deadly nightshades, which should be used only with extreme care. Belladonna is among the most toxic of all essential oils. Although it has a long history of benign use, including in cosmetics and medicines and as a surgical anesthetic, it has also been used as a deadly poison. Wolfsbane, which is also known as monkshood, is another deadly essential oil derived from a plant so poisonous that growers must avoid skin contact.

Before being crowned as king in 1040, Macbeth is said to have used nightshade to poison Danish invaders who landed on Scotland's shore. They demanded mead, which Macbeth laced with belladonna. Once the invaders had fallen into a stupor, Macbeth and his followers slaughtered them all.

Each of the body's cells contains electrons, which carry an electric charge and are affected by other sources of electricity. A number of medical treatments use electricity: think of the way a defibrillator can be used to restart the heart following cardiac arrest, and consider how electrotherapy is used in many beneficial ways, including stimulating the brain, helping injured muscles to heal, and improving blood flow.

Polarization is a process that separates positive and negative electrical charges within any object or energy form, including the body's cells and light. When light is polarized, its vibrations often occur in circular ellipses that can be used to promote healing within the body's tissues. Polarized light therapy is used in a number of medical applications, ranging from cosmetic procedures and treating skin disorders to providing relief from pain, speeding burn healing, treating ulcerated skin, and penetrating deep into joints to relieve pain.

Essential oils possess some of the same rotational properties as polarized light. Called dextrorotation and levorotation, these characteristics have a marked effect on the body's electromagnetic field. Researchers theorize that these properties contribute to the body's ability to heal itself in much the same way electric charges do.

In addition, essential oils have a profoundly positive effect on blood circulation. They can play an important role in carrying oxygen and vital nutrients to the body's tissues while aiding in the efficient disposal of the waste normal metabolism processes leave behind. By increasing blood flow, essential oils improve immune system efficiency and decrease blood viscosity, which in turn benefits the entire body, including the brain.

Though sweet-smelling and often used simply because their fragrances are so delightful, essential oils actually contain the most powerful chemicals plants are capable of synthesizing from the sun, the water, and the soil that nourishes them. Their molecular structures are incredibly complex and powerful, yet essential oils are easy and pleasurable to use.

While each essential oil is valuable on its own, they may be combined to form even stronger chemical compounds whose synergistic effects far surpass those of single oils. In contrast, very powerful oils and blends may be diluted to provide the correct dosage.

The Healing Power of Essential Oils

Many essential oils act as adaptogens, which are natural balancers. Adaptogens promote a balancing reaction in the body, which in turn can affect a multitude of the body's systems, including blood pressure, the autonomic nervous system, the endocrine system, and digestion.

Many essential oils are natural analgesics—substances that provide relief from pain by acting on the peripheral and ventral nervous systems. For instance, wintergreen essential oil contains between 85 and 99 percent methyl salicylate, which is the same active ingredient contained in aspirin. Before synthetic pain relievers were introduced in the 1920s, wintergreen and birch were considered to be the best remedies for pain; in fact, Native Americans used both plants before written records were ever kept.

Pain is characterized by a state of mental, emotional, or physical lack of well-being. While modern pharmaceuticals play an important role in managing pain, most of these drugs lack the power analgesic essential oils possess in that they often address physical pain only. Wintergreen essential oil is also known to bring about feelings of self-acceptance, and peppermint essential oil, which has been shown effective in blocking pain, is also renowned for its ability to promote an overall feeling of calm and well-being.

Doctors have battled against infections since the beginning of time, and some of the best tools in their arsenal are antiseptics, which are antimicrobial substances that reduce the potential for infection when applied to living tissues. Some antiseptics are also classified as germicides for their ability to destroy microbes, and others are antibacterial and inhibit microbial growth. Although most antiseptics manufactured today contain a variety of chemicals, antiseptic essential oils are completely natural. Some of the most powerful antiseptic essential oils include lavender oil, tea tree oil, and clove oil. There are many different ways to blend antiseptic essential oils to improve efficacy, and there are a variety of methods for using them, including infusing them in bathwater, applying them to minor wounds, or adding them to poultices or compresses.

Clove essential oil is so effective as an anti-inflammatory and analgesic that it has been approved for use as a dental anesthetic by the American Dental Association. It is excellent when included in mouthwash recipes, particularly if you suffer from sore, inflamed gums.

Inflammation is part of the body's defense system. This valuable immune response helps eliminate negative stimuli so the body's structures can begin to heal after an injury or following exposure to a harmful substance. When tissues become inflamed, redness, swelling, or pain can occur. When these symptoms last only for a short time, they are typically not harmful. When inflammation symptoms become chronic, they can begin to cause damage to the very same structures they are designed to protect. That's when minimizing inflammation becomes vital to continued health and well-being.

Many essential oils have anti-inflammatory properties. For example, thyme essential oil is a useful ingredient in blends designed to reduce muscle fatigue, while pure, unadulterated rose otto oil is effective in treating dry or inflamed skin and even in diminishing the appearance of broken capillaries.

Whether you are suffering from a skin condition, muscle soreness, chronic migraines, or other painful or irritating bodily conditions, there is a great likelihood that one or more of the many essential oils available will prove to be effective in alleviating your symptoms.

In addition to their therapeutic benefits, essential oils have many practical applications. For example, they can be used to create natural laundry detergents and nontoxic household cleaners. Some, such as citronella, make effective natural insect repellents. If you're looking for a way to reduce the amount of chemicals you use in your home, making your own products with essential oils is an excellent choice.

WHAT IS AROMATHERAPY?

Aromatherapy is a form of alternative medicine in which essential oils are used to positively influence a person's mind, bodily health, mood, or cognitive function. Though essential oils are at the heart of aromatherapy, complementary natural ingredients such as jojoba, herbs, hydrosols, mineral clays, and other substances are used as well.

Keep in mind that many items claiming to be aromatherapy products—including scented candles, perfume oils, and fragrance oils—actually contain synthetic ingredients. For any substance to be aromatherapeutic, it must be completely natural. Products with labeling such as "made with natural ingredients" or "made with essential oils" typically contain only small amounts of natural ingredients or essential oils, which is one reason many people choose to purchase their own essential oils and blend customized aromatherapy products at home. (See Chapter 3 for tips on blending).

*During the Dark Ages, aromatherapy was considered akin
to witchcraft, and aromatherapy practitioners were forced
underground. The Catholic church banned many natural remedies,
because believers viewed illness as a punishment from God. Followers were
instructed to pray and bleed themselves in hopes of obtaining a cure.*

The Science of Scent

The human sense of smell is about ten thousand times more powerful than other senses, and scent travels to the brain so rapidly that the mental or physical response to the fragrance an essential oil emits can be immediate. When you inhale an essential oil, its scent travels first through olfactory nerve cells inside the nose and into the larger olfactory system. The olfactory system then delivers the aroma to the olfactory bulb located inside the brain's limbic system, which serves as the seat of emotions and the originator of emotional behavior.

Depending upon which essential oil you are inhaling, you may feel a rapid release of mental strain or negative emotions, and you may feel muscle tension ease at the same time. You may feel more alert, excited, or engaged with your surroundings, and if the scent you are inhaling is a familiar one, you may rapidly access your collective unconscious and experience strong memories, particularly when those memories are closely associated with deeply emotional feelings.

The limbic system is, in turn, connected to the pituitary gland and the hypothalamus, which controls the release of hormones that affect one's nervous system, appetite, body temperature, concentration, and stress levels. Essential oils interact with the limbic system by providing input that activates the hypothalamus, instructing it to release neurochemicals to calm, relax, or stimulate the body. This is why aromatherapy can play such an important part in stress reduction, appetite control, increasing alertness, and much more. Whether essential oils are deeply inhaled or applied to the skin, the odor molecules travel straight to the appropriate limbic destination, where neurochemicals instruct the body to respond as desired.

Our individual senses of smell are a lot like fingerprints. Everyone smells different odors in a unique way, with the exception of identical twins, who have identical odor receptors and who process scents in exactly the same way. An essential oil that smells fantastic to one person may seem less than appealing to another.

Benefits of Aromatherapy

Many people find that aromatherapy helps bring about feelings of spiritual well-being. Frankincense is a classic example of an essential oil that has been used for centuries to add fragrance to sacred spaces such as churches, sanctuaries, and home meditation rooms. Diffusing frankincense and then taking long, slow breaths can help you focus as you embark upon any spiritual journey.

Essential oils have wonderfully positive effects on every level, with unique properties that enhance the body, mind, and spirit. Aromatherapy, when understood this way, is more than just the scientific application of essential oils to bring about beneficial changes in the physical realm; it is the creative use of essential oils to evoke positive changes on aesthetic and mystical levels as well.

CHAPTER TWO

Acquiring, Storing, and Using Essential Oils

HOW ARE ESSENTIAL OILS PRODUCED?

There are several different methods for extracting essential oils. Most extraction techniques rely on the fact that most essential oils blend well with other oils and fats, certain solvents, and even alcohol, but they do not mix with water. Over the years, herbalists and essential oils manufacturers have determined which methods work best for each plant, depending on that plant's unique chemical signature.

Expression

Expression is the most direct method for producing essential oils. In expression, the oil is simply pressed from the plant's seeds, flesh, or skins in a process similar to that used to press olive oil. This technique is primarily used to obtain essential oils from citrus peels: lemon, orange, grapefruit, and lime.

Solvents

Employing chemical solvents is the least natural method for extracting essential oils, and many professional aromatherapists shy away from oils produced in this manner. Although all the solvents used for extraction are supposed to be removed, some light chemical traces could potentially taint the finished product.

In this method, the plant from which the essential oil is sourced is dissolved in a chemical solvent: benzene, methylene chloride, and hexane are some common ones. As solvents have lower boiling points than essential oils, they are evaporated off, leaving the essential oil behind. A vacuum or centrifuge is typically employed to help separate the solvent from the essential oil.

Essential oils extracted with solvents are called "absolutes." Vanilla and jasmine essential oils are often produced this way as they cannot be distilled, and rose otto essential oil is often produced via solvent extraction because it is less expensive to produce when this method is used.

Hypercritical Carbon Dioxide

One of the newest methods for producing essential oils relies on plant interaction with carbon dioxide. Although producing essential oils this way is prohibitively expensive, the results are delightful. Essential oils produced using the carbon dioxide method smell almost exactly like the plants they were sourced from. Carbon dioxide becomes hypercritical—meaning it is neither a true gas nor a true liquid—at 33 degrees Celsius (91.4 degrees Fahrenheit). Extraction occurs rapidly with this method, and as carbon dioxide is inert, there is no chemical interaction between it and the plant from which the essential oil is being extracted.

Essential oils extracted with the help of carbon dioxide tend to be extremely high quality, and it is possible to find nearly any popular essential oil produced using this method. There are two different types to look for: CO_2 selects, and CO_2 totals.

CO_2 selects can be poured, just like other essential oils. They are typically a bit more viscous than oils produced using other methods; however, the plant's waxes, color compounds, and resins are left behind during processing.

CO_2 totals are extracted at higher pressures and contain the waxes, color compounds, and resins that are typically left behind during the essential oil manufacturing process. They usually have a thick, pasty consistency; however, they can be gently heated and blended with other essential oils and with carrier oils.

Steam Distillation

Most plants from which pure essential oils are obtained stand up well to the steam distillation process. In this simple procedure, freshly harvested plants are suspended above a vat of boiling water, and the steam emerging from the water extracts the oils from the plant. A vessel catches the rising steam, which is pushed through a tube before being cooled. The steam then condenses back into water, and as essential oils do not mix with water, the two substances separate. The essential oil is collected, and in many cases, the remaining water is collected as well, since it retains the fragrant character of the essential oil. This water is referred to as hydrosol and is often used in moisturizers, linen sprays, and simple perfumes.

Enfleurage

A very old method for producing essential oils that is rarely used in areas other than France, enfleurage is an expensive and complicated process. Whole blossoms are laid out on sheets coated with warm vegetable oil that in turn absorbs the oils from the flowers. As the oils are bled from the blossoms, exhausted flowers are replaced with fresh ones until all the oil has been infused with fragrance. The essential oil is then separated from the oil.

Hot enfleurage is the oldest-known method for extracting essential oils. This labor-intensive process involves melting fat (historically, pork lard or beef tallow) and stirring in botanical matter. As the flowers, leaves, and berries release their fragrance into the oil, spent botanicals are strained out and replaced with fresh ones. The resulting product is called enfleurage pomade. After essential oils have been extracted from the mixture with alcohol, the remaining fat is usually used to make soap, as it is normally quite fragrant.

ALL ESSENTIAL OILS ARE NOT CREATED EQUAL

There are many factors that determine essential oil quality. For example, plant species, extraction techniques, and even growing conditions, including soil quality, cloud cover, and environmental temperature, can affect the plants from which essential oils are extracted.

There are three characteristics crucial to determining the quality of a particular essential oil: grade, purity, and integrity.

Grade

When essential oils are produced, they are graded in the same way many other products are. The higher the grade is, the more costly the essential oil will be. For example, there are four grades of lemon essential oil, and at least twelve grades of lavender oil.

Grade is not necessarily an indicator that one type of essential oil is superior to another; in fact, the process of grading is quite subjective. Essential oils are very much like fine wines in that even seasoned experts have difficulty agreeing on favorites.

Often, grading is conducted as a method for specifying which types of essential oils are best for a specific use. For example, peppermint oil designated for delivery to candy manufacturers is graded differently that peppermint oil designated for aromatherapy use. Both grades are perfectly acceptable.

Once you have gained some experience in using essential oils on a regular basis, you will find that more expensive, higher-grade essential oil tends to have a more complex fragrance than lower grades do. As a rule, the more complex the fragrance, the more aromatic compounds an essential oil will contain.

Purity

When purchasing essential oils, particularly those you plan to use for aromatherapy, natural healing, or in cosmetics, it is vital that you look for pure essential oils. Unfortunately, some manufacturers and retailers dilute essential oils—particularly the most expensive ones—with similar-smelling essential oils, carrier oils, vegetable oils, alcohol, or solvents that might not even be derived from plants. When this is done, the resulting product is not capable of delivering the expected results.

Integrity

When essential oil manufacturers and retailers refer to a certain essential oil's integrity, they are referring to the fact that the oil comes from a single plant species, often from the same region, and often from the same harvest. In addition, integrity indicates that an essential oil is pure and natural.

Essential oils with integrity are not created in laboratories, nor are they created with other similar-smelling oils. An oil without integrity also might contain pure essential oils; for example, inexpensive citronella and lemongrass oils are often labeled as much more expensive lemon balm (Melissa) oil.

Detecting adulterated product is fairly simple. Oils that have been cut with alcohol tend to have an alcoholic odor; those that have been diluted with vegetable oils will separate when frozen. You can also detect carrier oil by placing a tiny drop of an essential oil on a sheet of white paper. If, after a few days, there is still an oily spot on the paper and the fragrance of the essential oil has evaporated, the oil you're testing has likely been diluted with a carrier oil.

BUYING AND STORING ESSENTIAL OILS

Purchasing your essential oils from a respected retailer is a good way to ensure that you are getting exactly what you need rather than a cheap, ineffective substitute. Dishonest sellers frequently label essential oils as "pure" when in fact exactly the opposite is true.

Selecting a Good Source

Until you gain the experience needed to discern high-quality essential oils from synthetics or cheap blends, the most important aspect of purchasing essential oils is the source. Some companies consistently sell high-quality essential oils, while others sell shoddy imitations. Though you might think that price is a good indicator of an essential oil's quality, this is not necessarily true.

Some companies use fancy packaging and advertise heavily; while a few of these companies do sell high-quality essential oils, many are more interested in selling nicely scented oils than therapeutic ones. At many retail locations with essential oils for sale, there is often nothing to rely on but labeling to determine whether an essential oil is worthwhile.

That said, you'll find essential oils as well as supplies (including diffusers and carrier oils) at natural food stores and on skin care and aromatherapy websites, as well as on auction sites and in large online marketplaces. Before making a purchase, do your best to learn about the seller's reputation. If you are buying essential oils online, be sure you know what you want, as you will not have an opportunity to sniff-test the oils before purchasing them. (See Additional Resources for a list of reputable retailers).

Price Differences

There is quite a bit of variability in the prices of essential oils, mostly because some are much more expensive to produce than others. For example, rose otto essential oil from Bulgaria is among the most costly; this is because it takes approximately six hundred pounds of rose petals to make just one ounce of pure rose otto essential oil. These delicate flowers must be cultivated with care and maintained with delicate precision. In Bulgaria, they are handpicked each morning before the sun's rays have a chance to release the fragrant oils of the roses into the air.

Jasmine essential oil is also very expensive, as it takes approximately twenty days of labor to produce a single ounce of jasmine oil. The delicate plants must be carefully tended and the tiny star-shaped flowers must be picked by hand—the exact opposite of what happens with an inexpensive essential oil such as mint. Mint grows in prolific abundance in many places and does not require much care. It can be harvested rapidly with farm equipment, and it contains an abundance of essential oil.

Purchasing cheap essential oils may cost you more in the long run. Low-quality oils are typically weaker than their high-quality counterparts, meaning you will end up using more to achieve the same effect. Taking this into consideration may help you save money over time.

Storing Essential Oils

Once you have chosen essential oils, it is vital that you store them properly. Always store essential oils in glass containers rather than in plastic ones. This is because many essential oils are so potent that they have a tendency to cause plastic to begin dissolving. Not only does this cause bottles to feel sticky, it can cause harmful chemicals to leach from the plastic into the oils. Store eyedroppers separately from essential oils, too, since their rubber bulbs and seals can be adversely affected by the oils just as plastic bottles can.

Properly stored, most essential oils will last for several years; in fact, several types are much like valuable wines in that they actually improve with age. Patchouli that has been properly stored for several years develops a rich fragrance that is nothing like fresh patchouli oil. Benzoin, clary sage, vetiver, and sandalwood also improve with age.

Citrus essential oils, including orange, lemon, and grapefruit, have a tendency to lose their potency over time. They last longer when refrigerated in dark-colored glass containers.

No matter what type of essential oils you prefer, keep them away from direct sunlight and store them well away from heat sources, since both sunlight and heat can cause them to lose their potency.

SAFETY TIPS AND PRECAUTIONS

While some essential oils are suitable for ingestion, others are safe only for topical application or for use in aromatherapy. Besides using the following general guidelines and precautions, keep all essential oils out of reach of children and pets, and never apply concentrated essential oils to mucous membranes or sensitive areas. Also, if you are allergic to a certain food, do not use any essential oils or carrier oils that come from the same plant as the allergen.

Conduct a Patch Test

Never assume that an essential oil has the same properties as the plant it came from. Even if you are familiar with certain plants and have used them in the past, conduct a patch test prior to using a new essential oil. To do this, apply a little diluted essential oil to your inner arm. Watch carefully for redness or irritation that develops either immediately or within as long as twenty-four hours; if it occurs, do not use the essential oil.

Your Skin and Essential Oils

Essential oils should rarely be applied neat (undiluted). Some, including those sourced from conifer and citrus trees, have strong caustic characteristics and come with warnings concerning dilution rates. Follow instructions carefully to avoid chemical burns.

People with sensitive skin or allergies must be doubly cautious when using essential oils. The least sensitive skin of the body is located on the soles of the feet, so using essential oils here will be less likely to produce irritation. Once you have used a particular oil on the soles of your feet without any problems, try using a small amount elsewhere on your body to determine if you can enjoy using it for more extensive topical application.

Everyone should use caution when applying essential oils to skin that has come into contact with cleaners or personal care products that contain synthetic chemicals. Many petrochemical-based products penetrate the skin and underlying fatty tissue; these chemicals can remain in the skin for days to weeks after application. When essential oils interact with these chemicals, nausea, skin irritation, headaches, and other unpleasant side effects can occur.

Essential oils can sometimes react with pollutants that have built up in the body from chemicals in the water we drink, the food we consume, and the environment we inhabit. If you experience any type of adverse reaction whatsoever, stop using essential oils and seek medical attention if needed.

Many people choose to undergo internal detoxification cleanses before starting an aromatherapy regimen. Simply doubling your water intake can help clear your body of toxins; drink purified water and avoid consuming water from plastic bottles.

Essential Oils and Sun Safety

Some essential oils, including bergamot, petitgrain, and most citrus oils, are phototoxic, meaning that skin irritation resembling a severe sunburn can result when these oils are applied to skin that is then exposed to sunlight. Do not apply them to skin that will be exposed to direct sunlight anytime within forty-eight hours of application.

In Case of an Accident Involving Essential Oils

To remove unwanted essential oils from the skin, cover the area with a carrier oil or an oil-based cleanser. Wash the area with soap and warm water, and repeat until you are certain the oil has been removed.

If essential oil gets into the eyes, flush them with vegetable oil or cold milk to dilute the oil, ensuring you remove contact lenses first if applicable. If stinging persists for more than a few minutes, seek medical attention.

Some essential oils, including mint, orange, and basil are meant to be consumed in small quantities; however, most are meant for external use only. If an essential oil is ingested accidentally, call your local poison control hotline.

TEN FREQUENTLY ASKED QUESTIONS ABOUT ESSENTIAL OILS

Q: *Is there a grading system for essential oils?*
A: No, there is no official grading system for essential oils.

Q: *Is it possible to burn essential oils for aromatherapy?*
A: It is best to use a diffuser, which gently warms the essential oils and releases them into the air.

Q: *How does the body absorb essential oils that have been applied topically?*

A: The skin is a porous organ that essential oils penetrate with ease. When the oils enter the bloodstream, they are distributed to the rest of the body.

Q: *Should pregnant women avoid essential oils?*

A: Always consult a physician and/or certified aromatherapist before using any type of essential oil during pregnancy or when breastfeeding.

Q: *What is an aromatherapy oil?*

A: An aromatherapy oil is one that can be purchased prediluted. These oils typically contain 98 percent carrier oil and 2 percent essential oil.

Q: *Do medical doctors ever use essential oils in treating patients?*

A: Many health professionals, including MDs, use essential oils as part of a holistic health practice.

Q: *What is the English method of aromatherapy?*

A: Historically, the English recommended that essential oils be applied topically. This is why topical application is also referred to as the English method.

Q: *Are essential oils ever administered intravenously?*

A: In some nations, medications containing essential oils are injected and administered intravenously. These methods are not accepted in the United States or Canada.

Q: *Why do many essential oils have long, complicated-looking names?*

A: Essential oils are labeled with their common names as well as with their Latin names, which are made up of the plant's genus and species.

Q: *How much essential oil does a typical bottle contain?*

A: Most essential oils are sold in 10-milliliter bottles. Some of the most popular, including mint, lavender, and orange essential oils, are also available in larger sizes, depending upon the distributor's standard practices.

CHAPTER THREE

Blending Essential Oils

HOW TO BLEND

Blending essential oils is not at all difficult, but there are a few things to keep in mind. First, consider what type of therapeutic action you hope to achieve with the essential oil. The best blends include oils that are enhanced when combined with others.

Second, consider the sequence of the essential oil blend. If you've ever cooked or baked, you know that ingredients often need to be added in a specific sequence for the best-tasting results. The same rule applies to essential oils. When you change the sequence, chemical reactions change, and the end results (including the fragrance) may vary from the original blend recipe.

Don't worry—if the thought of blending several different essential oils together is a daunting one, there are many carefully crafted essential oil blends on the market. The recipes included in this book are not at all difficult to make, though, so consider trying a few of them. Like cooking and baking, blending essential oils is something that becomes second nature over time if you do it often enough.

Fragrances were everywhere in the ancient world. In his book Natural History, *Pliny the Elder included lists of ingredients for creating customized perfumes along with some discussion of tools and techniques for blending fragrances.*

Two Rules for Blending Essential Oils

There are two basic rules to keep in mind when blending essential oils. While it is not necessary to commit these rules to memory, doing so will help you create better blends.

First, essential oils that have a lighter, thinner stream when poured are usually more aromatic (volatile) than those that are thicker. These oils have lighter, smaller molecules than their more viscous counterparts.

Second, the body absorbs light, small molecules faster than larger, heavier ones. The smaller the molecules a blend contains, the faster that blend is metabolized. The opposite is true of larger molecules. These are absorbed slowly and remain in the system longer.

These two rules matter because when you blend heavy molecules with lighter ones, they have a synergistic effect on one another, allowing for the lighter molecules to remain in the body longer. This is as important for creating therapeutic blends as it is for creating simple perfumes and aromatherapy blends designed to be diffused. In the perfume industry, the heavier oils, which act to stabilize the lighter, more volatile oils, are called fixatives or fixing oils. Sandalwood, myrrh, and ylang-ylang are excellent examples of fixing oils.

Classifying Notes

In aromatherapy, as you might suspect, the lightest oils are considered to be top notes. Here's where it gets tricky: the heaviest oils are considered to be middle notes. The ones in between are called base notes. The best blends contain various notes. Rather than blending three top notes or three middle notes together, it's best to select oils from each of the classifications. This strategy allows you to create balanced blends that are neither too heavy nor too volatile.

There is a second method for classifying essential oils that takes four characteristics into consideration rather than three: the personifier, the enhancer, the equalizer, and the modifier. When using this method for blending, following the same order each time will allow you to achieve consistent results.

The Personifier

Personifier oils should be used first and should comprise between 1 and 5 percent of the blend. These essential oils have strong, sharp aromas that linger, and they possess strong therapeutic action as well. Some personifiers are clove and clary sage.

The Enhancer

These oils are added second and should comprise between 50 and 80 percent of the blend. Tea tree and Melissa are examples of enhancers; they are dominant within the blend, and they have sharper aromas than the rest.

The Equalizer

Equalizer essential oils are added third and should comprise between 10 and 44 percent of the blend. They have bright fragrances, and they last a shorter amount of time than the other blends. Oregano is an excellent equalizer, and tea tree is sometimes used as an equalizer as well.

The Modifier

Modifier essential oils are added to the blend last, and should comprise between 5 and 8 percent of the mixture. These oils have mild aromas that add harmony to a blend. Rose otto and grapefruit are examples of modifier essential oils.

CARRIER OILS

Carrier oils are used to dilute essential oils and essential oil blends. Sweet almond, sesame, grape-seed, coconut, wheat germ, and sunflower oils are all examples of carrier oils; these can be used on their own or mixed together to create a texture and fragrance that is both pleasing and balanced. Passion-flower, avocado, and jojoba are also popular carrier oils.

Most therapeutic blends call for between twenty-five and thirty drops of essential oil to approximately half an ounce of carrier oil. Once you get a feel for blending, you'll find customizing blends is simple—it's basically a matter of preference.

Carrier oils should be of good quality, and it's best to use natural oils rather than synthetic ones. It makes no sense to purchase therapeutic-grade essential oils and use a low-grade gel, oil, or lotion to blend them.

Most oils made from flowers are volatile essential oils. Sunflower oil is a carrier oil that ranges from very pale yellow to dark amber in color. It contains large quantities of vitamins A, D, and E, which are wonderfully nourishing to the skin.

TEN BLENDING TIPS AND PRECAUTIONS

1. Store your blends correctly. Keeping them in dark-colored glass containers out of the sun and away from heat sources will help them retain stability and last longer.

2. Always leave a bit of air space in the bottle so the oil can breathe.

3. Use nonmetallic utensils for blending essential oils. Glass droppers and glass rods are best, as they will not leach chemicals into your blends.

4. When adding an essential oil or an essential oil blend to a carrier oil, prevent breakage by adding half the carrier oil to the storage container and then adding the essential oils. Next, add the second half of the carrier oil. Cap the mixture and tilt it gently back and forth to blend. This not only helps prevent accidents, it also ensures you get an even blend.

5. Many blends will keep for a long time, but anything more than six to nine months old containing citrus oils should not be applied to the skin. Making small batches will help prevent waste.

6. Use a wide variety of essential oils, and be certain to rotate those you use often to prevent sensitization and skin irritation. If you use a certain blend three days in a row, switch to a different blend for at least the next three days.

7. If you are allergic to a certain food, do not use any essential oils or carrier oils that come from the same plant that the allergen comes from.

8. Always follow instructions for diluting essential oils. These instructions should be located on the bottle.

9. Preblended essential oils are convenient, but they have a shorter shelf life than single pure essential oils. If you purchase these, buy small amounts and use them up quickly.

10. Less is more when it comes to blending and using essential oils. Applying too much of a certain oil can have an adverse effect. Start with a very small amount, particularly if you are new to aromatherapy.

HOW TO USE ESSENTIAL OILS

Before using any essential oils, it is vital that you have a clear purpose in mind. Do you hope to elevate your spirits, or would you like to relax? Perhaps you are looking for an effective natural remedy for a pounding headache, or maybe you'd like to blend some all-natural bath products. Whatever the case, always double-check that the oils you're using are right for the intended purpose.

Be certain to pay close attention to precautions for each essential oil before you begin. In addition, dilute the oils carefully, be informed about potential side effects associated with each oil, and watch for any adverse reactions.

Essential oils enter the body in three ways: inhalation, ingestion, or topical application. Within each of these methods, there are a variety of application methods that can be used. For example, you can massage essential oils into the skin, add them to a bath, spray them on, or apply them topically using compresses.

CHOOSING AN APPLICATION METHOD

The best application method for any given essential oil or blend depends on the essential oil itself as well as on the desired effect. The majority can be inhaled, many essential oils can be applied topically, and a few can be ingested.

To determine your application method, consider both the condition you wish to treat and the desired effect. For example, if you need to treat a wound, you'll most likely be applying essential oils topically. If you want to improve your mood, the most effective methods of application are topical application or inhalation. If you enjoy taking a hot bath and you add an aromatherapy blend to the water beforehand, you are applying the essential oil topically and inhaling it as its molecules rise up on the steam from your bath.

Inhalation

There are a variety of techniques for inhaling essential oils. They may be placed on a cloth and inhaled, added to a bowl of hot water and inhaled as steam, or inhaled directly from the bottle.

If placed on a cloth, simply hold the cloth near your nose and inhale deeply three times, exhaling fully between each inhale. Be sure not to touch the cloth to your face, particularly if the essential oil you are inhaling is not recommended for topical use.

If added to a bowl of hot water and inhaled as steam, start by heating the water to a fast simmer. Pour it carefully into a large bowl and add two to three drops of essential oil. Sit comfortably at a table with a towel draped around your neck. Next, place your face over the bowl and bring the towel up and over your head like a tent. Breathe slowly and deeply for a few moments. This method is wonderful for soothing congestion, particularly if you use eucalyptus essential oil.

To inhale an essential oil directly from the bottle, simply uncap the bottle and place it near your nose, being careful not to come into contact with your face. Breathe in and out three times, remembering to keep your breaths slow, deep, and even.

Inhaling essential oils into the lungs offers both psychological and physical benefits. Many relaxing oils, such as rose otto, chamomile, or sandalwood, can help alleviate anxiety, particularly when diffused. And achieving a pleasurable sense of emotional balance can have a therapeutic effect on the physical body, bringing particular relief to symptoms caused by excess stress.

The fragrance of an essential oil can stimulate the brain to trigger a specific reaction—such as relaxation or improved concentration—and the naturally occurring chemical constituents can provide a therapeutic benefit. For example, diffusing mandarin essential oil and inhaling deeply is an excellent way to ease stress.

Diffusion

There are a number of different essential oil diffuser models available, but most operate on the same basic principle. The diffuser is filled with water, a few drops of essential oil are added, and the diffuser is activated. As the water is heated, steam carrying tiny droplets of essential oil enters the room, and as you breathe, you slowly take in the essential oil. Some diffusers use a candle for heat, while others are electric.

Ingestion

Scented water made with distilled flowers or essential oils was used as a mouth rinse for centuries. Just before Marie Antoinette was executed in 1793, her servant was able to smuggle several toiletry items to her, including a vial of scented water with which to clean her teeth.

There are several essential oils that are safe to ingest. Keeping in mind that any essential oils used for ingestion must be therapeutic-grade, add a few drops of the selected essential oil to water or herbal tea for a refreshing and cleansing drink that can also be useful in treating various ailments. For example, lemon essential oil is a popular natural cold remedy and is also helpful for detoxifying the body. Just one or two drops of lemon essential oil mixed with a glass of fresh water can help soothe indigestion. Grapefruit essential oil is an appetite stimulant when ingested, and it can also help the body's lymphatic system to function better. Grapefruit oil is best taken just one or two drops at a time and mixed with cool water.

Of all the essential oils that are suitable for ingestion, peppermint essential oil is probably the most popular. A common ingredient in candies and chewing gum, this refreshing oil has also been used for centuries to treat cold symptoms, nausea, and indigestion. Though you may feel tempted to try consuming straight peppermint oil, doing so could cause discomfort. Mix a drop or two with a glass of water or herbal tea for best results.

Topical Application

When an essential oil is applied to the skin, it eventually makes its way into the bloodstream. As it travels through the body, it can ease pain, soothe indigestion, and push toxins from the body's cells. Essential oils and the carrier oils used to dilute them are often beneficial to the skin and hair, which makes them ideal for addition to a daily beauty routine. As essential oils are powerful and highly concentrated, it is important to dilute them properly before application. Grape-seed oil, sweet almond oil, and apricot kernel oil are some of the most popular carrier oils; all of these nourish and moisturize the skin.

Essential oils are also natural deodorizers and some, such as tea tree oil, are renowned for their powerful cleansing and skin toning properties. As part of an everyday routine, these oils are not only pleasurable to use, they are also excellent replacements for costly commercial cosmetic products.

Baths, massages, compresses, and facial steams are all wonderful to begin with, but when you add essential oils, they take on an added aesthetic dimension that makes even the simplest of beauty routines feel like a luxurious spa experience. When used in applications such as these, essential oils go a long way. Adding just a few drops of grapefruit oil or lavender oil to your favorite skin-softening carrier oil and then sprinkling a small amount of that mixture into a warm bath can help you soak away the cares of a stressful day.

Ancient Romans made a fine art of bathing. Scented water made with rose petals and other flowers was such a decadent delight that eventually scented water fountains were installed in public places for the refreshment of spectators.

Other Methods

If none of the preceding methods will work for you or if you find yourself in a pinch, there are a few other ways to use essential oils.

Humidifier

Fill your humidifier with clean filtered water. Place a few drops of essential oil on a cloth, and put the cloth in front of the steam vent. This method works very much like a diffuser, but it often propels essential oil molecules farther. Do not put essential oil directly into your humidifier. It will only float on top of the water, and it may cause damage to the machine.

Dry Evaporation

Place several drops of essential oil on a cotton ball or a folded tissue or cloth, and simply allow it to evaporate. You can inhale deeply if you like, or simply keep the cotton ball in your immediate vicinity—for example, next to your computer while working.

Instead of using chemical-laden room sprays, enjoy a dose of aromatherapy while freshening the air. Fill a clean sprayer (that has never contained chemicals) with filtered water, and add a few drops of your favorite essential oil. Shake thoroughly to blend, and spritz away!

TEN TOOLS TO GET YOU STARTED

As someone who is new to essential oils, you don't need a diploma or even a certificate to start reaping the rewards of using essential oils on a regular basis. Here are ten tools to get you started.

1. Precision droppers ensure you get the correct dosage and don't waste any essential oil. Purchase a few droppers so you'll always have one on hand when you need it.

2. Dark-colored glass containers protect your blends from excessive light and ensure they will retain their efficacy as long as possible. Blue, green, or brown glass bottles are best. Collect a variety of sizes and shapes; as you become more comfortable with making your own recipes, these will provide safe storage.

3. Nonmetallic tools are best for mixing essential oils. You can find glass rods online for only a few dollars.

4. Simple glass bowls from your kitchen are perfect for creating fragrant aromatherapy blends at first, but it's nice to have bowls dedicated for use with essential oils.

5. A glass funnel makes pouring blends into bottles simple.

6. Keep at least one type of carrier oil on hand, and consider purchasing a few more, if only to determine which you prefer.

7. A diffuser is an excellent item to have on hand, as diffusion is one of the easiest methods for enjoying aromatherapy. Many people who enjoy using essential oils on a regular basis keep a few diffusers in different locations around the house and office.

8. A glass spray bottle or two allows you to create fresh-smelling, healthy room sprays.

9. You'll need a place to keep your essential oils. While an upper shelf might work well, the small bottles are easily misplaced or knocked over, making an essential oil portfolio a nice item to have around. These padded portfolios protect essential oils and help keep them organized.

10. Labels are useful for marking blends and avoiding confusion. Consider keeping a small notebook with basic information about the essential oils you have on hand and information about the blends you have created, particularly as you continue to expand your knowledge base.

PART TWO

Oils, Recipes, and Remedies

CHAPTER FOUR

Nature's Apothecary

There are hundreds of varieties of essential oils available, each with a unique chemical signature, and each with the ability to promote well-being. The essential oils included in this chapter have been widely researched and are well-known for both their efficacy and safety. Choose therapeutic-grade essential oils if possible, and check each oil's Latin name before purchase to ensure you are getting the benefits you desire.

Allspice   *Pimenta officinalis*

....

DESCRIPTION

Warm and spicy, this cocoa-brown essential oil has a thin consistency and is used as a middle note in aromatherapy blends.

ORIGIN

Central America, Greater Antilles, Southern Mexico

PROPERTIES

Analgesic, anesthetic, antibacterial, antifungal, antioxidant, antiseptic, antiviral, aphrodisiac, carminative, stimulant

APPLICATION

Dilute three drops of allspice essential oil in an ounce of carrier oil before use. It is suitable for topical application and diffusion only, as it can irritate the nasal lining if directly inhaled.

PRIMARY USES

Eases stiffness, arthritis, and rheumatism pain; soothes gastric and muscular cramps; calms coughs and bronchitis; alleviates nausea and indigestion; reduces nervousness; eases tension; elevates mood.

BLENDS WITH

Bay, bergamot, black pepper, carrot seed, clove, geranium, ginger, lavender, neroli, patchouli, orange, ylang-ylang

SAFE USE

Do not take allspice essential oil internally. In addition, ensure it is diluted prior to inhalation or topical application, as it is a strong mucus membrane and dermal irritant.

Angelica Root *Angelica arcangelica*

DESCRIPTION

Sometimes referred to as "female ginseng," angelica root essential oil has a thin consistency and is pale yellow in color. It is used as a base note in aromatherapy.

ORIGIN

Canada, Hungary, Siberia

PROPERTIES

Antibacterial, antifungal, antispasmodic, carminative, depurative, diaphoretic, digestive, diuretic, emmenagogue, expectorant, febrifuge, nervine, stimulant, stomachic, tonic

APPLICATION

Dilute angelica root essential oil 50:50 before use. It may be applied topically, diffused, inhaled, or ingested.

PRIMARY USES

Brightens dull skin; alleviates psoriasis symptoms; eliminates water retention, detoxifying the body; soothes gout; fights coughs and colds; alleviates premenstrual symptoms and menstrual cramps.

When used in meditation, angelica root essential oil opens up a connection with the divine and encourages the release of repressed memories and negative emotions.

BLENDS WITH

Cedar, chamomile, clary sage, German chamomile, grapefruit, juniper, lemon, oakmoss, orange, patchouli, Roman chamomile, tangerine, vetiver

Angelica root essential oil is phototoxic; avoid exposure to the sun for twenty-four hours after use. In addition, using angelica root essential oil prior to outdoor activities is not recommended, as it sometimes attracts insects.

Historically, angelica root was used to combat plague. Once called "oil of angels," it was said to be of divine origin. As it blooms around the time of the feast of the Archangel Michael, it was named in his honor.

Basil *Ocimum basilicum*

....

DESCRIPTION

A thin, clear-colored oil, basil essential oil has a pleasant spicy scent that is reminiscent of licorice. When used in aromatherapy, it is considered a top note.

ORIGIN

France, Hungary, United States, Vietnam

PROPERTIES

Antibacterial, antidepressant, antiseptic, antispasmodic, carminative, cephalic, digestive, emmenagogue, expectorant, febrifuge, nervine, stimulant, stomachic, tonic

APPLICATION

Basil essential oil is wonderfully versatile. It may be taken internally, used in cooking, applied topically, and inhaled or diffused.

PRIMARY USES

Relaxes muscles; soothes body aches and bug bites; alleviates rheumatism symptoms; eases colds, coughs, headaches, and bronchitis; stimulates digestion; prevents flatulence; alleviates gout; repels insects.

Basil essential oil promotes clearheadedness and stimulates the mind. When used in meditation, it can promote trust, openness, and enthusiasm while releasing stagnant energy.

BLENDS WITH

Bergamot, citronella, citrus, clary sage, geranium, hyssop, lemongrass, mandarin, orange, peppermint, rosemary, spearmint, tangerine

SAFE USE

Dilute basil essential oil 50:50 prior to topical application or diffusion. Pregnant women and those with epilepsy should avoid basil essential oil. It may cause skin irritation.

Bergamot *Citrus bergamia*

....

DESCRIPTION

This golden-green essential oil has a thin consistency and a fresh, citrus-like aroma with floral undertones. When used in aromatherapy blends, it is considered a top note.

ORIGIN

Mediterranean countries, United States

PROPERTIES

Analgesic, antibacterial, antidepressant, antiseptic, antispasmodic, astringent, carminative, deodorant, digestive, diuretic, expectorant, febrifuge, laxative, sedative, stimulant, tonic, vermifuge, vulnerary

APPLICATION

Dilute by adding one part bergamot essential oil to four parts carrier oil. This essential oil is suitable for direct inhalation and ingestion, and for diffusion and topical application when diluted.

PRIMARY USES

Alleviates painful skin conditions, including acne, abscesses, psoriasis, and boils; relieves itchy skin; balances oily skin; comforts coughs; reduces cold symptoms; soothes insect bites and cold sores; prevents halitosis; promotes feelings of peaceful relaxation; alleviates stress and anxiety.

When used in meditation, bergamot essential oil can support healthful detoxification from drug and alcohol addiction, and aids in smoking cessation.

BLENDS WITH

Allspice, basil, cardamom, chamomile, citronella, citrus, clary sage, clove, coriander, cypress, frankincense, geranium, German chamomile, ginger, grapefruit, helichrysum, holy basil, jasmine, juniper, lavender, lemon, lemongrass, marigold, Melissa, myrrh, myrtle, neroli, nutmeg, oakmoss, orange, palmarosa, palo santo, patchouli, petitgrain, Roman chamomile, rosemary, rose otto, sandalwood, Scots pine, vetiver, violet, yarrow, ylang-ylang

SAFE USE

Bergamot essential oil is generally considered safe; however, it is not recommended for use with children younger than five years old. Applying bergamot essential oil without diluting it first can cause skin irritation, and repeated use can lead to contact sensitization. It is extremely phototoxic; direct sunlight and UV light should be avoided for as long as seventy-two hours after use.

Bergamot gives Earl Grey tea its distinctive flavor. It's also a very popular perfume additive: approximately a third of all colognes and half of all perfumes contain bergamot.

Black Pepper *Piper nigrum*

DESCRIPTION

Black pepper oil has a complex, green fragrance and does not irritate the eyes or cause sneezing, as ground black peppercorns often do. This crisp, fresh-smelling essential oil has a thin consistency and is considered a middle note when used in aromatherapy.

ORIGIN

China, India, Indonesia, Madagascar, Malaysia

PROPERTIES

Analgesic, antifungal, anti-catarrhal, anti-inflammatory, antiseptic, aphrodisiac, expectorant, laxative, stimulant (circulatory, digestive, nervous), warming

APPLICATION

Black pepper essential oil may be diffused or directly inhaled. It may also be applied topically or used as a dietary supplement. Dilute black pepper essential oil 50:50 before diffusing or applying topically.

PRIMARY USES

Improves circulation; soothes muscle soreness; alleviates joint, arthritis, and rheumatism pain; relieves nausea and indigestion; prevents flatulence; boosts metabolism; stimulates endocrine system.

When used in aromatherapy and meditation, it alleviates worry, soothes anxiety, and aids in releasing negativity and recognizing self-worth. Black pepper essential oil is also excellent for culinary use; a single drop goes a long way.

Allspice, cardamom, clary sage, cypress, frankincense, grapefruit, helichrysum, jasmine, juniper, lavender, lemon, lemongrass, lime, mandarin, myrtle, orange, palo santo, peppermint, Peru balsam, rosemary, rose otto, sandalwood, tangerine, vetiver, yarrow

SAFE USE

Black pepper essential oil is generally considered safe. It can cause severe skin irritation if used undiluted.

While traveling on pilgrimages, Indian monks consumed several peppercorns each day. They believed the peppercorns would give them greater physical endurance to see their journeys through.

Blue Cypress *Callitris intratropica*

....

DESCRIPTION

Blue cypress essential oil has a thin consistency and a clear to pale yellow color; occasionally it has a blue tint. Its distinct notes of lemon and cedar give it a fresh, sweet scent.

ORIGIN

Australia

PROPERTIES

Anti-inflammatory, antiviral, insecticide, stimulant

APPLICATION

Blue cypress essential oil should be diluted 50:50 before topical or diffuser use. It may be directly inhaled neat.

PRIMARY USES

Alleviates mild pain and skin rashes, including eczema; relieves viral symptoms, flu, and colds; repels insects; relieves abdominal cramps; promotes healthy digestion.

Blue cypress is balancing and grounding. When used during meditation, it helps release mental irritation and restlessness. It also promotes clear thinking.

BLENDS WITH

Blood orange, cedar, eucalyptus, laurel, rosemary, sandalwood

SAFE USE

Never apply blue cypress essential oil to skin without diluting it, as irritation can occur.

Cardamom *Elettaria cardamomum*

A sweet and spicy oil with a clear color and a thin consistency, cardamom essential oil is considered a middle note when used for aromatherapy.

ORIGIN

Guatemala, India, Sri Lanka

PROPERTIES

Antiseptic, antispasmodic, carminative, cephalic, digestive, diuretic, laxative, nervine, stimulant, stomachic

APPLICATION

Cardamom essential oil is extremely versatile. It may be taken internally, inhaled directly, or blended 50:50 with a carrier oil and diffused or applied topically.

PRIMARY USES

Relieves abdominal discomfort, heartburn, vomiting, and indigestion; eliminates halitosis and flatulence; alleviates headaches, sciatica, and sinus infections.

Cardamom essential oil has a sweet, uplifting fragrance that refreshes the mind. When used in meditation, it helps alleviate stress, release trauma, and helps one to accept new ideas.

BLENDS WITH

Bay, bergamot, black pepper, caraway, cinnamon, clary sage, clove, coriander, fennel, ginger, grapefruit, jasmine, lemon, lemongrass, mandarin, neroli, orange, palmarosa, patchouli, petitgrain, sandalwood, vetiver, ylang-ylang

SAFE USE

Cardamom essential oil is generally considered safe. Irritation can result if applied to the skin undiluted.

Carrot Seed *Daucus carota*

....

DESCRIPTION

Also known as wild carrot, carrot seed essential oil has a yellow-gold color and a thin to medium consistency. Its fragrance is woody and earthy, and many consider its smell unpleasant on its own. When used in aromatherapy, it is considered a middle note.

ORIGIN

France, Hungary, India

PROPERTIES

Antiseptic, carminative, depurative, diuretic, emmenagogue, hepatic, stimulant, tonic, vermifuge

APPLICATION

Blend carrot seed essential oil in a 50:50 ratio with a carrier oil prior to use. It may be ingested as a dietary supplement, diffused or directly inhaled, or applied topically.

PRIMARY USES

Alleviates pain from sunburn, rheumatism, and psoriasis; reduces appearance of wrinkles; tones oily skin; decreases itchiness caused by eczema; detoxifies the liver; prevents water retention.

When used in aromatherapy and for meditation, it aids in the release of negativity and promotes self-acceptance. Carrot seed essential oil is excellent for cultivating gratitude.

BLENDS WITH

Allspice, cedarwood, cinnamon, citrus, geranium, nutmeg

Carrot seed essential oil is generally regarded as safe. No special precautions are indicated.

In ancient times, carrot seeds were believed to have contraceptive properties. Hippocrates and other physicians prescribed carrot seeds to those seeking birth control.

Catnip *Nepeta cataria*

....

DESCRIPTION

A pale yellow to orange oil with a medium consistency, catnip essential oil has a lovely herbaceous aroma with a minty undertone. It is considered a middle note when used in aromatherapy blends.

ORIGIN

Canada, United States

PROPERTIES

Anesthetic, anti-inflammatory, antirheumatic, antispasmodic, astringent, carminative, diaphoretic, insecticide, sedative, tonic

APPLICATION

Dilute catnip essential oil 50:50 in a carrier oil before topical application. It may be diffused or inhaled directly.

PRIMARY USES

Alleviates arthritis, rheumatism, and minor injury pain; repels insects.

Nepetalactone, catnip's active constituent, has been found to be more effective than DEET at repelling mosquitoes and other bugs. As could be expected, cats enjoy catnip essential oil; dab a tiny amount on a favorite toy for maximum fun.

BLENDS WITH

Grapefruit, lavender, lemon, marjoram, orange, peppermint, rosemary, spearmint

SAFE USE

Pregnant women should avoid contact with catnip essential oil, as should babies and very young children.

Chamomile *Matricaria recutita*

DESCRIPTION

Chamomile essential oil has a deep blue color, a thin consistency, and a sweet, herbaceous fragrance with fruity undertones. When used for aromatherapy, it is considered to be a middle note.

ORIGIN

Afghanistan, Canada, Europe, Iran, United States

PROPERTIES

Analgesic, anesthetic, anti-infectious, anti-inflammatory, antioxidant, antispasmodic, decongestant, digestive tonic, hormone-like, relaxant

APPLICATION

Chamomile essential oil may be used neat. It is suitable for topical application, direct inhalation, diffusion, or ingestion.

PRIMARY USES

Soothes itchy skin; eases chronic tension; relieves headaches and migraines; eliminates insomnia; alleviates premenstrual tension and menopausal symptoms; promotes feelings of calm; dissipates anger.

BLENDS WITH

Angelica root, benzoin, bergamot, citrus, clary sage, clove, cypress, eucalyptus, frankincense, geranium, helichrysum, jasmine, lavender, lemon, lemon tea tree, marjoram, Melissa, mountain savory, myrrh, myrtle, neroli, nutmeg, oakmoss, palmarosa, patchouli, rosemary, rose otto, sage, sandalwood, spearmint, spruce, tea tree, yarrow, ylang-ylang

SAFE USE

Chamomile essential oil is generally considered safe. People with sensitive skin may suffer irritation following topical application.

Cinnamon   *Cinnamomum verum*

....

DESCRIPTION

A medium-bodied oil with a golden to yellow-brown color, cinnamon essential oil has a strong cinnamon scent. When used in aromatherapy applications, it is considered a middle note.

ORIGIN

Sri Lanka

PROPERTIES

Antibacterial, anticoagulant, antidepressant, antifungal, anti-infectious (urinary, intestinal), anti-inflammatory, antimicrobial, antioxidant, antiparasitic, antiseptic, antiviral, astringent, warming

APPLICATION

Dilute cinnamon essential oil 20:80 with a carrier oil (one part cinnamon oil to four parts carrier oil). It may be diffused, applied topically, or used as a dietary supplement.

PRIMARY USES

Alleviates urinary and intestinal discomfort; stimulates the immune system, circulatory system, and libido; relieves coughs; alleviates cold and flu symptoms; soothes inflammation; increases circulation; mitigates diabetes symptoms.

Cinnamon essential oil is believed by some to attract wealth. When used in meditation, it aids in transformative thought, releases anger and frustration, and helps alleviate addictions of all types.

BLENDS WITH

Cardamom, carrot seed, frankincense, jasmine, lemon tea tree, mandarin, orange, palo santo, rosemary, rose otto, tangerine, tea tree, ylang-ylang

Cinnamon essential oil is extremely strong and can cause serious skin irritation if applied neat. Do not directly inhale cinnamon essential oil, as it can burn delicate nasal passages.

Cinnamon is one of the oldest-known essential oils. It was recorded in the Ebers Papyrus, *one of the earliest Egyptian medical texts, which dates to approximately 1550 BCE and contains more than seven hundred remedies for everything from asthma to indigestion—along with instructions for properly embalming the deceased to ensure they enjoy a happy afterlife.*

Citronella *Cymbopogon nardus*

....

DESCRIPTION

A thin, clear oil with a slightly fruity, sweet scent and a strong citrus characteristic, citronella essential oil is considered a top note when used in aromatherapy blends.

ORIGIN

Java, Sri Lanka, Vietnam

PROPERTIES

Analgesic, antibacterial, antifungal, antiseptic, antispasmodic, astringent, deodorant, diaphoretic, diuretic, febrifuge, insecticide, stimulant, tonic

APPLICATION

Dilute citronella essential oil 50:50 with a carrier oil before diffusing or applying topically. It may be inhaled directly and is suitable for use as a dietary supplement.

PRIMARY USES

Repels insect; alleviates cold and flu symptoms; relieves muscle pain, fatigue, headaches, and migraines; treats acne and oily skin.

BLENDS WITH

Basil, bergamot, cedar, citrus, geranium, holy basil, rosemary, sandalwood, Scots pine

SAFE USE

Women who are pregnant should avoid contact with citronella essential oil. Those with heart disease should avoid it, too, as it can increase heart rate. Do not apply to skin without diluting, as irritation can result.

Clary Sage *Salvia sclarea*

DESCRIPTION

This light golden-yellow oil has a thin to medium consistency and an invigorating herbaceous aroma, with subtle notes of fruit and earth. It is considered a middle note when used in aromatherapy blends.

ORIGIN

Bulgaria, France, United States

PROPERTIES

Antibacterial, antidepressant, antiseptic, antispasmodic, aphrodisiac, astringent, carminative, deodorant, digestive, euphoric, sedative, stomachic, vulnerary

APPLICATION

Dilute clary sage essential oil 50:50 with a carrier oil before diffusing or applying externally. It may be directly inhaled and is suitable for use as a dietary supplement.

PRIMARY USES

Alleviates premenstrual symptoms and menstrual cramps, premenopausal symptoms, and hormonal imbalances; promotes healthful cholesterol levels; relieves insomnia; improves circulation; relieves tired eyes when added to eye wash; alleviates bronchitis symptoms; boosts mood.

Clary sage essential oil quiets the mind and promotes a gentle sense of euphoria. When used in meditation, it promotes enhanced creativity and increases focus. It is also used to enhance the ability to enjoy vivid dreams.

BLENDS WITH

Angelica root, basil, bay, bergamot, black pepper, cardamom, chamomile, clove, coriander, cypress, frankincense, geranium, German chamomile, grapefruit, helichrysum, holy basil, hyssop, jasmine, juniper, lavender, lemongrass, lemon tea tree, lime, mandarin, Melissa, myrtle, neroli, nutmeg, oakmoss, orange, palmarosa, patchouli, petitgrain, Roman chamomile, rosemary, rose otto, sandalwood, Scots pine, spikenard, spruce, tangerine, tea tree, vetiver, yarrow, ylang-ylang

SAFE USE

Clary sage essential oil is generally recognized as safe. It can irritate the skin if applied undiluted, and it should never be applied undiluted to the eye area. Women who are pregnant should avoid clary sage oil, as should very small children.

Clary sage gets its name from the nickname medieval authors gave it: "clear eye," for its ability to heal vision problems. It was also used, like chamomile, as a substitute for hops in ale production, and it was added to wine to heighten the drinker's sense of intoxication.

Clove *Syzygium aromaticum*

....

DESCRIPTION

Often called clove bud essential oil, clove essential oil has a spicy, warming scent and a golden to yellow-brown hue. It has a medium, slightly oily consistency, and when used in aromatherapy blends, clove essential oil is considered a middle note.

ORIGIN

Indonesia, Madagascar, Sri Lanka

PROPERTIES

Analgesic, antiaging, antibacterial, anticlotting, antifungal, anti-inflammatory, antimicrobial, antioxidant, antispasmodic, antiseptic, antiviral, carminative, expectorant, insecticide, stimulant

APPLICATION

Dilute clove essential oil 20:80, adding one part essential oil to four parts carrier oil. Clove essential oil may be diffused, applied topically, or ingested.

PRIMARY USES

Numbs arthritis and rheumatism pain; soothes insect bites and bee stings; relieves inflammation and digestive problems, including diarrhea, nausea, and vomiting.

Clove essential oil is used by naturopaths to treat lupus, hepatitis, viral infections, cataracts, skin cancer, and thyroid disorders. When it is used in aromatherapy and for meditation, clove bud essential oil aids in the release of negativity and the acceptance of self-worth.

BLENDS WITH

Allspice, bay, bergamot, cardamom, chamomile, clary sage, geranium, German chamomile, ginger, grapefruit, helichrysum, jasmine, lavender, lemon, lemon tea tree, mandarin, myrrh, myrtle, orange, palmarosa, patchouli, petitgrain, Roman chamomile, rose otto, sandalwood, spikenard, tangerine, tea tree, vanilla, wintergreen, ylang-ylang

SAFE USE

Clove essential oil is extremely powerful. Never inhale it neat, as it can irritate the nasal passages, and do not apply it to skin undiluted, as serious skin irritation can result.

This essential oil is an anticoagulant; it can enhance the effects of aspirin, heparin, warfarin, and other blood thinners.

Cypress   *Cupressus sempervirens*

DESCRIPTION

Pale yellow in color, with a thin consistency, cypress essential oil has an evergreen aroma with hints of wood and herbs. When used in aromatherapy blends, it is considered a middle note.

ORIGIN

France, Morocco, Spain

PROPERTIES

Antibacterial, anti-inflammatory, antiseptic, antispasmodic, astringent, deodorant, diuretic, emmenagogue, expectorant, febrifuge, insecticide, sedative, tonic

APPLICATION

Dilute cypress essential oil 50:50 with a carrier oil before applying topically or diffusing.

PRIMARY USES

Slows perspiration; eases hemorrhoid discomfort, menorrhagia, and menstrual cramps; improves circulation; eases varicose vein discomfort; treats muscle spasms; tones excessively oily skin; detoxifies the lymphatic system; reduces water retention.

When used in aromatherapy or for meditation, cypress essential oil has a calming, grounding effect. It promotes feelings of total well-being and assists in discernment while alleviating fear of the unknown.

BLENDS WITH

Benzoin, black pepper, cedarwood, chamomile, citrus, clary sage, eucalyptus, frankincense, geranium, German chamomile, ginger, grapefruit, helichrysum, jasmine, juniper, lavender, lemongrass, lemon tea tree, marigold, myrrh, palo santo, peppermint, petitgrain, Roman chamomile, rose otto, rose geranium, Scots pine, spikenard, tea tree, yarrow, ylang-ylang

SAFE USE

Women who are pregnant should avoid cypress essential oil. While it is generally recognized as safe, it can cause skin irritation if applied neat.

The word cypress is derived from the Greek term sempervirens, which means "to live forever." The Greeks used cypress to carve statues of their deities.

Douglas Fir *Pseudotsuga menziesii*

DESCRIPTION

Douglas fir essential oil has a complex evergreen fragrance. It is a medium-bodied oil and is considered a middle note when blended for aromatherapy.

ORIGIN

Canada, France, United States

PROPERTIES

Antifungal, antiseptic, antitussive, calmative, disinfectant, expectorant, nervine, pectoral, stomachic, tonic, vasodilator

APPLICATION

Dilute Douglas fir essential oil 50:50 with a carrier oil before topical application or diffusion. It may be directly inhaled neat or diluted.

PRIMARY USES

Soothes cold, flu, and bronchitis symptoms; eases muscle soreness and arthritis and rheumatism pain.

When used in aromatherapy or meditation, Douglas fir essential oil alleviates anxiety and soothes nervous tension. It has a grounding, stabilizing influence and aids in promoting feelings of physical and emotional security.

BLENDS WITH

Bergamot, cistus, fir needle, galbanum, jasmine, lavender, lemon, marjoram, rosemary, Scots pine

SAFE USE

Women who are pregnant should avoid Douglas fir essential oil. It is not suitable for internal use and may cause skin irritation if applied undiluted. It is toxic to cats.

Echinacea *Echinacea purpurea* or *E. angustifolia*

DESCRIPTION

Echinacea essential oil is light in color, with a thin to medium consistency. It has a sweet, floral aroma and may be used as a middle note in aromatherapy blends.

ORIGIN

Austria, Canada, Russia, United States

PROPERTIES

Antibiotic, anti-inflammatory, antimicrobial, antiviral, diaphoretic, immune stimulant

APPLICATION

Echinacea essential oil may be applied topically, directly inhaled, diffused, or ingested.

PRIMARY USES

Relieves tension, useful in treating tension headaches; strengthens the immune system; relaxes the mind; eases cold and flu symptoms; soothes insect bites, minor burns, and minor wounds; speeds healing of rashes, eczema, and other skin irritation, including acne; improves digestion; eases flatulence.

BLENDS WITH

Ginger, lemon tea tree, niaouli, tea tree, thyme, yarrow

SAFE USE

Echinacea essential oil is generally considered safe. Anyone taking immune-suppressing medication (particularly transplant patients) should avoid contact as it could interfere by stimulating the immune system and causing an unwanted immune response. Women who are pregnant or nursing may use echinacea essential oil topically, but they should not ingest it.

Eucalyptus *Eucalyptus globulus*

DESCRIPTION

There are over seven hundred eucalyptus species, many of which are used in the production of eucalyptus essential oil. Only a handful of these species are effective when used in aromatherapy. Of these, *Eucalyptus globulus* is most popular, and it should not be confused with *E. radiata* (sometimes nicknamed black peppermint essential oil), *E. citriodora* (lemon eucalyptus essential oil), or any other type of eucalyptus essential oil. Eucalyptus essential oil has a fresh woody, earthy fragrance, with a strong medicinal aroma and a thin consistency. When used in aromatherapy, it is considered a top note.

ORIGIN

Australia, Brazil, Spain

PROPERTIES

Antiaging, antibacterial, antifungal, anti-infectious, anti-inflammatory, antirheumatic, antiseptic, deodorant, expectorant, insecticide, mucolytic

APPLICATION

Eucalyptus essential oil should be diluted 50:50 with a carrier oil prior to use. It is suitable for direct inhalation, diffusion, and topical application. *Eucalyptus globulus* is suitable for ingestion; other forms of eucalyptus essential oil are not.

PRIMARY USES

Soothes arthritis, rheumatism, and muscle pains; eases sinusitis, coughs, bronchitis, cold and flu symptoms, and ear inflammation; combats candida, chicken pox, and measles symptoms; reduces acne; cleanses minor wounds; eases diabetes symptoms; boosts immune system.

Eucalyptus essential oil is used in manufacturing, as a fragrance for cosmetics and perfumes, and in antiseptics, ointments and liniments, cough drops, toothpaste, and other products. Some dentists use eucalyptus oil as a solvent for root canal fillings. It is also often used for treating chronic obstructive pulmonary disease (COPD) and cancer.

In addition, eucalyptus essential oil is useful as an insect repellent and as a natural flea deterrent. When properly diluted, it can be used on pets as well as humans. It makes a fantastic addition to massage oils and lotions, household cleaning products, and bath products, including shampoos and conditioners. When inhaled, eucalyptus essential oil can be used to promote emotional well-being, and during meditation it is useful for focusing on relationships.

BLENDS WITH

Blue cypress, cedar, chamomile, cypress, geranium, German chamomile, ginger, grapefruit, juniper, lavender, lemon, lemon tea tree, marjoram, myrrh, oakmoss, orange, peppermint, Roman chamomile, rosemary, Scots pine, spearmint, tea tree, thyme, wintergreen

SAFE USE

Eucalyptus oil must be diluted prior to use. Add one part essential oil to four parts carrier oil before adding to any recipe or applying topically. Only use therapeutic-grade eucalyptus oil, and conduct a patch test using diluted eucalyptus essential oil prior to applying any product that contains it.

When Jean Valnet, MD, ran out of antibiotics during World War II, he discovered that eucalyptus oil was effective in killing almost three-quarters of staph bacteria in the air. You, too, can squash bacteria with this powerful essential oil: if you're beginning to catch a cold, try inhaling steam from a basin filled with hot water and a few drops of eucalyptus essential oil. You may just stop that cold in its tracks.

Fir Needle   *Abies balsamea*

DESCRIPTION

Sometimes referred to as silver fir, fir needle essential oil is slightly yellow with a thin, slippery texture. It is considered a middle note when used in aromatherapy blends and has a wonderfully fresh, woody fragrance with sweet, earthy undertones.

ORIGIN

Bulgaria, France, Germany

PROPERTIES

Analgesic, antiseptic, antitussive, astringent, deodorant, expectorant, stimulant, tonic

APPLICATION

Dilute fir needle essential oil 50:50 with a carrier oil before topical application or diffusion. It may be directly inhaled neat.

PRIMARY USES

Soothes burns, cuts, and other minor wounds; alleviates muscle aches and soothes arthritis pain; eases bronchitis, coughs, sore throat, and sinusitis.

Fir needle essential oil is a natural deodorizer. When used in aromatherapy or for meditation, fir needle essential oil promotes relaxation, calm, and a feeling of overall well-being.

BLENDS WITH

Benzoin, cistus, Douglas fir, juniper, lavender, lemon, marjoram, orange, rosemary, Scots pine, tangerine

Fir needle essential oil is generally recognized as safe. It may cause skin irritation if applied undiluted. It is not intended for internal use. This essential oil is toxic to cats.

Frankincense *Boswellia carterii*

DESCRIPTION

Frankincense essential oil has an irresistible woody, balsamic fragrance, a light yellow color, and a thin consistency. When used in aromatherapy blends, it is considered a base note.

ORIGIN

Europe, India, North Africa

PROPERTIES

Analgesic, antifungal, anti-inflammatory, antioxidant, antiseptic, astringent, carminative, digestive, diuretic, expectorant, sedative, tonic, vulnerary

APPLICATION

Frankincense essential oil may be directly inhaled or blended 50:50 with a carrier oil before being diffused or applied topically. It is also suitable for use as a dietary supplement.

PRIMARY USES

Boosts immune system and combats infections; alleviates coughs, sore throat, strep, pneumonia, and staph symptoms; reduces stress and nervous tension; boosts mood.

When used for aromatherapy or during meditation, frankincense essential oil provides an uplifting, centering effect that promotes a deep sense of inner calm. Many believe frankincense opens a pathway directly to the divine; it is a favorite for diffusing during prayer sessions.

BLENDS WITH

Bergamot, black pepper, chamomile, cinnamon, clary sage, cypress, geranium, German chamomile, ginger, grapefruit, jasmine, lavender, lemon, mandarin, marigold, Melissa, myrrh, neroli, orange, palmarosa, patchouli, petitgrain, Roman chamomile, rosemary, rose otto, sandalwood, Scots pine, spikenard, tangerine, vetiver, ylang-ylang

Frankincense essential oil is generally recognized as safe. It can cause skin irritation if applied undiluted.

The uses and benefits frankincense provides have been well known for at least five thousand years. It is mentioned in the Bible fifty-two times, and was very popular with the Egyptians, who used it for stomach ailments, skin care, and incense. Kohl, which was used as eyeliner, was made from frankincense.

Galbanum *Ferula galbaniflua*

DESCRIPTION

Galbanum essential oil is clear, with a thin consistency. When used in aromatherapy blends, it is considered a top note. It is highly prized for its spicy, balsamic aroma.

ORIGIN

Iran, Turkey

PROPERTIES

Analgesic, anti-inflammatory, antimicrobial, antiseptic, antispasmodic, balsamic, carminative, digestive, diuretic, emmenagogue, expectorant, hypotensive, restorative, tonic

APPLICATION

Galbanum essential oil may be diluted; however, it is one of the few essential oils that may be used neat. It may be diffused, directly inhaled, applied topically, and ingested as a dietary supplement.

PRIMARY USES

Alleviates pain; treats cuts, boils, and minor wounds; improves circulation; aids digestion; eases inflammation; softens scar tissue; tones skin; smoothes appearance of wrinkles; combats stress and nervous tension.

When used in aromatherapy or meditation, galbanum essential oil aids in centering and grounding the mind, letting go of old ideas, and embracing new ways of thinking.

BLENDS WITH

Benzoin, Douglas fir, geranium, ginger, lavender, oakmoss, Scots pine, spruce

Galbanum essential oil is generally considered safe and is approved for use as a food flavoring agent and food additive by the US Food and Drug Administration (FDA).

Geranium *Pelargonium graveolens*

Geranium essential oil has a thin consistency and ranges in color from clear to light amber. It has a fresh floral aroma with a hint of fruit, and is considered a middle note when used in aromatherapy blends.

ORIGIN

Egypt, France, Italy, Spain

PROPERTIES

Analgesic, antibacterial, antidepressant, antidiabetic, anti-inflammatory, antiseptic, astringent, deodorant, diuretic, insecticide, regenerative, sedative, styptic, tonic, vasoconstrictor, vermifuge, vulnerary

APPLICATION

Dilute geranium essential oil 50:50 with a carrier oil before diffusing or topical application. It may be directly inhaled or ingested as a dietary supplement, and it is excellent for baths and room sprays.

PRIMARY USES

Alleviates anxiety and stabilizes emotions; heals broken capillaries, bruises, and circulatory disorders; eliminates fluid retention; soothes insect bites, stings, burns, and minor wounds; relieves sore throat and lymphatic congestion.

When used in aromatherapy or for meditation, geranium essential oil lifts the spirit while easing nervous tension. It can help alleviate fear concerning abandonment or commitment, and it can help promote self-acceptance.

BLENDS WITH

Allspice, basil, bergamot, carrot seed, chamomile, citronella, clary sage, clove, cypress, eucalyptus, frankincense, galbanum, German chamomile, ginger, grapefruit, helichrysum, holy basil, hyssop, jasmine, juniper, lavender, lemon, lemongrass, lemon tea tree, mandarin, Melissa, myrrh, neroli, nutmeg, orange, palmarosa, palo santo, patchouli, peppermint, petitgrain, Roman chamomile, rosemary, rose otto, sandalwood, spikenard, tangerine, tea tree, vetiver, ylang-ylang

SAFE USE

Women who are pregnant should avoid geranium essential oil. It may cause skin irritation, particularly if applied undiluted.

German Chamomile *Matricaria chamomilla*

....

DESCRIPTION

Often referred to as blue chamomile due to its deep blue color, German chamomile essential oil has a thin consistency and a sweet, herbaceous aroma with fruity undertones. It is considered a middle note when used in aromatherapy blends.

ORIGIN

Afghanistan, Bosnia, Canada, Europe, Hungary, Iran, United States

PROPERTIES

Analgesic, anesthetic, anti-infectious, anti-inflammatory, antioxidant, antispasmodic, antitumoral, decongestant, digestive tonic, hormone-like, relaxant

APPLICATION

German chamomile essential oil may be used neat. It is suitable for direct inhalation, diffusion, topical application, and ingestion.

PRIMARY USES

Promotes healing of broken capillaries, bruises, and minor wounds; soothes insect bites, muscle spasms, arthritis pain, and sprains; alleviates nausea, stress, and nervous tension; aids sleep.

When used in aromatherapy or for meditation, German chamomile essential oil can help calm feelings of irritation and anger while promoting peace, clarity, and patience.

BLENDS WITH

Angelica root, benzoin, bergamot, citrus, clary sage, clove, cypress, eucalyptus, frankincense, geranium, helichrysum, jasmine, lavender, lemon, lemon tea tree, marjoram, Melissa, mountain savory, myrtle, neroli,

nutmeg, palmarosa, patchouli, rosemary, rose otto, sage, sandalwood, spearmint, spruce, tea tree, yarrow, ylang-ylang

SAFE USE

Women who are pregnant should avoid German chamomile essential oil
and other chamomile products. It can cause skin irritation.

*German chamomile was one of the herbs listed in Europe's first guide
to medicine, Pedanius Dioscorides' De Materia Medica—the first
known standard reference book of herbal treatments, written in 78 CE.*

Ginger   *Zingiber officinale*

....

DESCRIPTION

There are more than 1,200 species of ginger; of these, *Zingiber officinale* is best suited to medicinal and internal use. It is an excellent essential oil for blending with others; for example, when blended with juniper, it provides a powerful detoxifying effect. Ginger essential oil has a warm, spicy aroma with delightful notes of earth and wood. It has a thin consistency and is typically steam distilled. When used in aromatherapy, it can be used as a middle or base note.

ORIGIN

India, Jamaica, Nigeria, Sri Lanka

PROPERTIES

Anesthetic, anticoagulant, anti-inflammatory, digestive, expectorant, laxative, stimulant, tonic, warming

APPLICATION

Ginger essential oil should be diluted 50:50 with a carrier oil prior to use. It is suitable for direct inhalation, diffusion, and topical application. It is also suitable for ingestion and is useful for culinary applications.

PRIMARY USES

Reduces congestion and respiratory infections; eases motion sickness, indigestion, nausea, and diarrhea; soothes angina and sore throats; prevents scurvy.

Ginger essential oil can help kick car sickness. For humans, apply a few drops of ginger oil to a cloth and inhale deeply. For dogs, place a few drops of diluted ginger oil on a front paw, where the scent of the oil will stay close to the pet's nose.

Ginger essential oil is uplifting and energizing; in addition, it has an aphrodisiac effect when used in aromatherapy. Its sweet, spicy aroma enhances feelings of vitality and promotes a feeling of physical well-being while enhancing energy. When used in meditation, it can help promote self-confidence and provide motivation to transform ideas into realities.

BLENDS WITH

Allspice, bergamot, cardamom, cedar, clove, coriander, cypress, echinacea, eucalyptus, frankincense, galbanum, geranium, grapefruit, jasmine, juniper, lemon, lemongrass, lemon tea tree, lime, mandarin, myrtle, neroli, oakmoss, orange, palmarosa, patchouli, Peru balsam, rose otto, sandalwood, tea tree, vetiver, ylang-ylang

SAFE USE

Ginger oil can be taken internally, applied externally, and enjoyed in aromatherapy blends. Always dilute it before use, adding one part essential oil to one part carrier oil. Use only therapeutic-grade ginger essential oil, and conduct a patch test with diluted essential oil prior to applying it topically.

Ginger essential oil is generally regarded as safe. However, it is photosensitive and direct exposure to sunlight within twenty-four hours of use may cause dermatitis. In addition, it is an anticoagulant and it may enhance the action of blood thinners, including aspirin, heparin, warfarin, and others. Consult your physician if you use blood thinners and you would like to use ginger essential oil.

Grapefruit *Citrus paradisi*

··

DESCRIPTION

Grapefruit essential oil is a favorite not just for its delightful scent, but for its ability to help ease water retention and congestion. Grapefruit essential oil is derived from *Citrus paradisi* fruit peels. Both pink and white grapefruit essential oils are available, with the pink variety normally being more sweetly scented than the white. Its sweet, tangy, tart citrus fragrance blends beautifully with other essential oils, including white pine oil and frankincense oil. This essential oil is cold pressed or expressed. It has a thin consistency, and when used in aromatherapy, it is considered a top note.

ORIGIN

United States, West Indies

PROPERTIES

Antidepressant, antiseptic, antitumoral, cleansing, detoxifying, disinfectant, diuretic, fat dissolving, metabolic, stimulant, tonic

APPLICATION

Grapefruit essential oil should be diluted 50:50 with a carrier oil prior to use. It is suitable for direct inhalation, diffusion, topical application, and ingestion.

PRIMARY USES

Treats headaches, anxiety, and depression; eases Alzheimer's symptoms; combats obesity; reduces appearance of cellulite; eliminates water retention and puffy skin; cleanses liver, kidneys, lymph system, and vascular system; boosts mood; promotes physical energy; repels insects.

Grapefruit essential oil is particularly effective against fleas, and if you have horses, it helps repel flies. It can be used in formulating nontoxic household products, massage oils, lotions, and bath products, including shampoos and conditioners.

When used in meditation, it aids in releasing confusion, clearing mental chatter, and relieving feelings of sadness and tension. It is also known for its ability to bring clarity and a renewed sense of spiritual purpose.

BLENDS WITH

Angelica root, bergamot, black pepper, cardamom, catnip, chamomile, clary sage, clove, cypress, eucalyptus, fennel, frankincense, geranium, German chamomile, ginger, hyssop, jasmine, juniper, lavender, lemon, lemongrass, mandarin, myrrh, neroli, orange, palmarosa, palo santo, patchouli, peppermint, Roman chamomile, rosemary, sandalwood, Scots pine, tangerine, thyme, vetiver, yarrow, ylang-ylang

SAFE USE

Conduct a patch test before using grapefruit essential oil on your skin. Dilute it by adding one part essential oil to one part carrier oil prior to topical use. Also, grapefruit essential oil is phototoxic. Avoid exposing skin to direct sunlight for twenty-four hours after application. Like other citrus essential oils, grapefruit oil may be ingested. Take only one to two drops at a time, blended in a glass of water or herbal tea. Grapefruit essential oil has a very short shelf life in comparison with most other essential oils. Buy it in small quantities and use it up within six months of purchase.

While grapefruit essential oil is beneficial to dogs and horses, it is toxic to cats. Cats will not normally be attracted to this oil; however, if a cat ingests it accidentally, contact your veterinarian.

If you open a bottle of white wine or champagne and the taste doesn't seem quite right, try adding a single drop of grapefruit essential oil to the bottle to completely transform its taste. This is especially fantastic in Sauvignon Blanc.

Helichrysum Helichrysum italicum

DESCRIPTION

With a fresh, earthy fragrance and a thin consistency, helichrysum essential oil has a light yellow color. It is considered a base when used in aromatherapy blends.

ORIGIN

Bosnia, France, Italy, Spain

PROPERTIES

Antibacterial, anti-inflammatory, antimicrobial, antioxidant, antispasmodic, astringent, diuretic, expectorant, febrifuge, hepatic, stimulant

APPLICATION

Helichrysum essential oil may be diluted 50:50 or used neat. It is suitable for direct inhalation, diffusion, topical application, and ingestion.

PRIMARY USES

Speeds the healing of bruises, burns, and minor wounds; alleviates muscle aches and pains; soothes pain from sprains and strains; softens dry skin; soothes sunburns; reduces appearance of scars and stretch marks; slows or stops minor bleeding; soothes coughs; reduces fevers; calms nerves; relieves tension.

When used in aromatherapy or for meditation, helichrysum essential oil helps remove emotional blocks and promote perseverance. It is ideal for anyone suffering from mental stress or anxiety.

BLENDS WITH

Bergamot, black pepper, chamomile, citrus, clary sage, clove, cypress, geranium, German chamomile, juniper, lavender, lemon tea tree, neroli, oakmoss, oregano, palmarosa, Roman chamomile, rosemary, rose otto, tea tree, vetiver, wintergreen, ylang-ylang

Helichrysum essential oil is generally considered safe, and the FDA recognizes it as a food additive.

Holy Basil   *Ocimum sanctum* and *O. tenuiflorum*

DESCRIPTION

Also known as tulsi, holy basil essential oil has a pale yellow color and a thin consistency. It is considered a top note when used in aromatherapy blends, and has a strong, warm, spicy aroma.

ORIGIN

India, Sri Lanka

PROPERTIES

Adaptogen, antibacterial, antidepressant, antioxidant, antiviral, carminative, diuretic, expectorant, immunomodulator

APPLICATION

Diffuse, directly inhale, apply topically, or use holy basil essential oil sparingly in herbal tea. Extreme dilution is required, usually at a ratio of one to three drops holy basil oil per ounce of carrier oil.

PRIMARY USES

Supports respiratory and digestive health; energizes and stimulates the mind; enhances focus; eliminates stress and eases anxiety.

When used in aromatherapy or for meditation, holy basil essential oil enhances mental clarity while promoting spiritual purity.

BLENDS WITH

Bergamot, citronella, citrus, clary sage, geranium, hyssop, jasmine, oakmoss, rose otto

Holy basil essential oil is extremely powerful and can cause severe skin irritation if applied without dilution. Women who are pregnant or nursing should not use this essential oil.

In India, holy basil is sacred to the Hindu deity Vishnu. It is used in morning prayers, and strings of beads made from the plant's stems are used during meditation. Ancient Ayurvedic texts mention it as a remedy for snakebites and scorpion stings.

Hyssop *Hyssopus officinalis*

DESCRIPTION

With a fresh, slightly sweet aroma bearing undertones of fruit, earth, and wood, hyssop essential oil is clear, with a thin consistency. When used in aromatherapy blends, it is considered a middle note.

ORIGIN

France, Hungary, Spain

PROPERTIES

Antibacterial, antiseptic, antispasmodic, antiviral, astringent, carminative, cephalic, digestive, diuretic, expectorant, febrifuge, hypertensive, sedative, tonic, vermifuge, vulnerary

APPLICATION

Hyssop essential oil should be diluted, using one part hyssop essential oil to four parts carrier oil. It is suitable for diffusion, direct inhalation, topical application, and ingestion.

PRIMARY USES

Restores appetite after illness; raises low blood pressure; alleviates anxiety, fatigue, and nervous tension; combats respiratory infections, congestion, and viral infections.

When used in aromatherapy or for meditation, hyssop essential oil stimulates creativity, aids in understanding one's spiritual purpose, and releases self-doubt and self-judgment.

Basil, bay, clary sage, geranium, grapefruit, holy basil, lavender, lemon, mandarin, myrtle, orange, rosemary, sage

SAFE USE

Hyssop essential oil is generally regarded as safe. The FDA has approved it for use as a food additive.

Jasmine   *Jasminum officinale* or *J. grandiflorum*

....

DESCRIPTION

Though jasmine blossoms are pure white, jasmine essential oil is a deep gold to amber color. It has a medium consistency and is considered a middle note when used in aromatherapy blends.

ORIGIN

Egypt, France, India, Italy

PROPERTIES

Analgesic, anti-inflammatory, aphrodisiac, carminative, emmenagogue, expectorant, tonic

APPLICATION

Jasmine essential oil may be used neat for topical application, diffusion, or direct inhalation.

PRIMARY USES

Eases anxiety; boosts mood; soothes respiratory illnesses, including congestion; alleviates premenstrual symptoms; promotes hormonal balance; relieves skin conditions, including acne and eczema.

When used in aromatherapy or for meditation, jasmine essential oil aids in bringing about emotional balance, alleviating fear, and promoting euphoria. Jasmine essential oil is also a noted aphrodisiac.

BLENDS WITH

Bergamot, black pepper, cardamom, chamomile, cinnamon, clary sage, clove, coriander, cypress, Douglas fir, frankincense, geranium, German chamomile, ginger, grapefruit, holy basil, lemon, mandarin, myrrh, neroli, orange, palmarosa, patchouli, Peru balsam, petitgrain, Roman chamomile, rose otto, sandalwood, spearmint, tangerine, vetiver, ylang-ylang

Do not ingest. Women who are pregnant should not use jasmine essential oil.

Jasmine's nickname is "Queen of the Night." The plant's blossoms are most fragrant during the evening, so they are normally harvested just after the sun goes down.

Juniper *Juniperus communis*

··

DESCRIPTION

Often called juniper berry essential oil, juniper essential oil has a distinctive woody fragrance with a hint of sweetness. It has a thin consistency and is clear; when used in aromatherapy blends, it is considered a middle note.

ORIGIN

Bulgaria, Canada, France, Nepal, United States

PROPERTIES

Analgesic, antimicrobial, antiseptic, antispasmodic, astringent, digestive, diuretic, sedative

APPLICATION

Dilute juniper essential oil 50:50 with a carrier oil. It may be diffused, directly inhaled, applied topically, or ingested.

PRIMARY USES

Purifies air; repels insects; soothes skin conditions, including acne, eczema, and dermatitis; softens scar tissue; promotes nerve regeneration after injury; relieves gout; reduces water retention.

When used for aromatherapy or during meditation, juniper essential oil aids in releasing suppressed anger and negativity.

BLENDS WITH

Angelica root, black pepper, cedarwood, clary sage, cypress, elemi, eucalyptus, fir needle, geranium, ginger, grapefruit, helichrysum, lavender, lemongrass, lemon tea tree, mandarin, myrrh, neroli, oakmoss, orange, palmarosa, peppermint, petitgrain, rosemary, sage, Scots pine, spikenard, tangerine, tea tree, wintergreen

Juniper essential oil is generally regarded as safe, and is approved as a food additive by the FDA. Juniper berries have been used in culinary applications for millennia and are the primary flavoring agent in gin.

Lavender   *Lavandula angustifolia*

··

DESCRIPTION

Lavender essential oil is by far one of the most popular aromatherapy oils available, and its benefits are nearly endless. Lavender essential oil is a floral, but its fragrance is not sweet like most other florals. Instead, it is fresh and strongly herbal, with camphor undertones. This essential oil has a thin consistency, and is typically steam distilled. When used in aromatherapy, it can be a top or middle note.

ORIGIN

Bulgaria, France, Ukraine, United States

PROPERTIES

Analgesic, antibacterial, anticonvulsant, antifungal, antiseptic, antispasmodic, antitumoral, vasodilator, vermifuge

APPLICATION

Lavender essential oil may be used neat. It is suitable for direct inhalation, diffusion, topical application, and ingestion.

PRIMARY USES

Soothes insomnia, nervous tension, and premenstrual symptoms; treats skin conditions, including acne and excess oil on the skin; reduces blood pressure and cholesterol; treats allergies and asthma; soothes bruises and burns; eases headaches; combats mild bacterial and fungal infections, including swimmer's ear and athlete's foot; repels insects.

Lavender essential oil can be used to formulate nontoxic household products, lotions, massage oils, and bath products. It can also be used to promote a sense of calm and balance, as well as to relax the mind and ease feelings of anger and frustration. When used for meditation, it promotes feelings of clarity and invites greater intuition.

Allspice, bergamot, black pepper, catnip, cedar, chamomile, clary sage, clove, cypress, Douglas fir, eucalyptus, fir needle, frankincense, galbanum, geranium, German chamomile, grapefruit, helichrysum, hyssop, juniper, lemon, lemongrass, lemon tea tree, lime, mandarin, marigold, marjoram, Melissa, myrrh, myrtle, neroli, nutmeg, oakmoss, orange, palmarosa, palo santo, patchouli, peppermint, Peru balsam, petitgrain, Ravensara, Roman chamomile, rosemary, rose otto, sage, sandalwood, Scots pine, spearmint, spikenard, spruce, tea tree, thyme, valerian, vetiver, yarrow

SAFE USE

Conduct a patch test before using lavender essential oil on your skin. This is one of the few essential oils that's considered safe to apply undiluted; however, some individuals can suffer skin irritation when the oil is applied topically.

Lavender essential oil can be poisonous if ingested; when teas and extracts are taken orally, they can cause constipation, headaches, and changes in appetite. As lavender essential oil has a relaxing effect, it may increase drowsiness when used in conjunction with sedatives.

Native to the Mediterranean region, lavender was used as a bath additive throughout Persia, Rome, and Greece. Its Latin name comes from lavare, *which means "to wash."*

Lemon *Citrus limon*

DESCRIPTION

Lemon essential oil has a fragrance much like that of fresh lemon zest. It is pale to deep yellow in color and has a thin consistency. When used in aromatherapy blends, lemon essential oil is considered a top note.

ORIGIN

Italy, United States

PROPERTIES

Antibacterial, antifungal, anti-inflammatory, antimicrobial, antirheumatic, antiseptic, antispasmodic, astringent, carminative, digestive, diuretic, laxative

APPLICATION

Dilute lemon essential oil 50:50 with a carrier oil. It may be diffused, directly inhaled, applied topically, or ingested.

PRIMARY USES

Repels insects; aids the digestive process; soothes indigestion; detoxifies the liver; improves circulation; soothes insect bites; tones oily skin; smoothes appearance of wrinkles.

Lemon essential oil is excellent for use in natural household cleansers and bath products. It also makes a wonderful addition to insect repellents for humans, dogs, and horses. When used in aromatherapy or for meditation, lemon essential oil can aid in improving concentration. It uplifts the mind and body while releasing negativity and promoting a sense of joy.

BLENDS WITH

Angelica root, benzoin, bergamot, black pepper, cardamom, catnip, chamomile, clove, Douglas fir, eucalyptus, fennel, frankincense, fir needle, geranium, German chamomile, ginger, grapefruit, hyssop, jasmine, juniper, lavender, lemongrass, lemon tea tree, mandarin, myrrh, myrtle, neroli, oakmoss, orange, palmarosa, palo santo, peppermint, petitgrain, Roman chamomile, rosemary, rose otto, sage, sandalwood, Scots pine, spearmint, spikenard, tangerine, tea tree, vetiver, wintergreen, ylang-ylang

SAFE USE

Lemon essential oil is generally regarded as safe. Use caution when applying it topically, as it is phototoxic and can cause skin irritation. Avoid exposure to direct sunlight for at least twenty-four hours after application.

Lemon oil is often used to protect unsealed wood and provide a natural sheen. Guitars, violins, and other stringed instruments are often treated with lemon essential oil.

Lemongrass *Cymbopogon flexuosius*

....

DESCRIPTION

Lemongrass essential oil is yellow in color and has a thin consistency. With
a fresh, earthy, lemon scent, it is considered a top note when used in aromatherapy blends.

ORIGIN

Madagascar, Nepal, Sri Lanka

PROPERTIES

Analgesic, antibacterial, antifungal, anti-inflammatory, antimicrobial, antioxidant, antiparasitic, antiseptic, antiviral, astringent, deodorant, digestive,
febrifuge, insecticide, sedative, tonic

APPLICATION

Dilute lemongrass essential oil 20:80, using one part essential oil to four parts
carrier oil. It may be directly inhaled, diffused, applied topically, or ingested.

PRIMARY USES

Speeds healing of ligament and tendon injuries; repels insects; aids sedation; dilates blood vessels to promote healing and improve circulation;
promotes lymphatic flow.

When used in aromatherapy or for meditation, lemongrass essential oil
clears the mind and heightens psychic awareness. It aids in the release
of regret and resentment while promoting feelings of hope, courage,
and optimism.

BLENDS WITH

Basil, bergamot, black pepper, cardamom, clary sage, coriander, cypress,
geranium, ginger, grapefruit, juniper, lavender, lemon, lemon tea tree,

marjoram, orange, palmarosa, patchouli, rosemary, tea tree, thyme, vetiver, wintergreen, ylang-ylang

Lemongrass essential oil may cause skin irritation if applied undiluted.

Lemon Tea Tree *Leptospermum petersonii*

....

DESCRIPTION

Lemon tea tree essential oil has a yellow tint and a thin consistency. It has a sharp citrus fragrance and is considered a top note when used in aromatherapy blends.

ORIGIN

Australia

PROPERTIES

Antiseptic, antimicrobial, carminative, sedative

APPLICATION

Lemon tea tree essential oil may be used neat or diluted 50:50 with a carrier oil. It is suitable for direct inhalation, diffusion, and topical application.

PRIMARY USES

Repels insects; soothes arthritis and rheumatism pain; calms itchy skin; heals minor burns and small wounds; relieves cold and flu symptoms; aids sedation.

When used in aromatherapy or for meditation, lemon tea tree essential oil promotes relaxation and an overall sense of peace and well-being.

BLENDS WITH

Clove, cypress, eucalyptus, geranium, ginger, juniper, lavender, lemon, mandarin, orange, peppermint, rosemary, Scots pine, thyme

Lemon tea tree essential oil can cause dermal sensitization; apply only as needed. It is not recommended for ingestion.

During World War II, tea tree producers and tea tree farm workers were granted exemption from military service until enough essential oil had been harvested. The oil was then issued to soldiers and sailors for treatment of topical infections and minor wounds.

Lime *Citrus aurantifolia*

··

DESCRIPTION

Lime essential oil has a light green color and a thin consistency. When used in aromatherapy blends, it is considered a top note; it has a fresh, sweet, citrus scent that many find irresistible.

ORIGIN

India, Malaysia, United States

PROPERTIES

Antiseptic, antibacterial, antiviral, aperitif, astringent, disinfectant, febrifuge, restorative, styptic, tonic

APPLICATION

Dilute lime essential oil 50:50 with a carrier oil. It may be directly inhaled, diffused, applied topically, or ingested.

PRIMARY USES

Eases anxiety; freshens air; disinfects household surfaces; relieves acne; cleanses oily hair; reduces appearance of wrinkles; combats viral and bacterial infections.

When used in aromatherapy or during meditation, lime essential oil promotes improved concentration and uplifts the mind. It aids in releasing negativity and cellular memory after physical or emotional trauma.

BLENDS WITH

Black pepper, cedar, citrus, clary sage, ginger, lavender, myrtle, neroli, nutmeg, oakmoss, vanilla, ylang-ylang

SAFE USE

Lime essential oil can be phototoxic; avoid exposure to direct sunlight for at least twenty-four hours after use.

Mandarin *Citrus reticulata*

....

DESCRIPTION

Mandarin essential oil has a greenish orange hue and a thin consistency. It has a sweet, citrusy fragrance, and when used in aromatherapy blends, it is considered a top note.

ORIGIN

Brazil, Italy, Spain, United States

PROPERTIES

Antiseptic, antispasmodic, carminative, digestive, diuretic, hypnotic, laxative, lymphatic stimulant, sedative, tonic

APPLICATION

Dilute mandarin essential oil 50:50 with a carrier oil. It may be directly inhaled, diffused, applied topically, and ingested.

PRIMARY USES

Eases constipation; relieves fluid retention; aids digestion; stops hiccupping; alleviates acne and other skin disorders; reduces appearance of scars and stretch marks.

Mandarin essential oil is an excellent addition to skin care products for the face and body. When used in aromatherapy or for meditation, mandarin essential oil promotes feelings of relaxation and well-being. It eases nervous tension and is excellent for diffusing around edgy toddlers.

BLENDS WITH

Basil, black pepper, cardamom, cinnamon, clary sage, clove, frankincense, geranium, ginger, grapefruit, hyssop, jasmine, juniper, lavender, lemon, lemon tea tree, myrrh, neroli, nutmeg, palmarosa, palo santo, patchouli, petitgrain, rosemary, rose otto, sandalwood, tea tree, valerian, vetiver, ylang-ylang

SAFE USE

Mandarin essential oil is generally considered safe. It can be phototoxic for those with sensitive skin; avoid direct sun exposure for twenty-four hours after application if your skin is sensitive.

Marigold *Calendula officinalis*

....

DESCRIPTION

Also known as calendula essential oil, marigold essential oil is thick and deep yellow, with a sticky consistency and a very strong musky fragrance. It is suitable for use as a base note in aromatherapy applications.

ORIGIN

Canada, Egypt, Southern Europe, United States

PROPERTIES

Anti-inflammatory, antioxidant, antispasmodic, emmenagogue, sudorific, tonic

APPLICATION

Marigold essential oil may be applied neat or diluted 50:50 with a carrier oil prior to use. It is suitable for topical application, direct inhalation, diffusion, and ingestion.

PRIMARY USES

Soothes acne symptoms, itchy skin, and rashes, including eczema and psoriasis; heals minor burns, bruises, and cuts; reduces appearance of scars and stretch marks; treats insect bites, including bee stings; repels insects.

Historically marigold essential oil was used as a food dye; it adds a slight floral flavor to icings and baked goods.

BLENDS WITH

Arnica, bergamot, cypress, frankincense, laurel, lavender

SAFE USE

Marigold essential oil is generally considered safe. It is one of the few essential oils that's suitable for use in preparations intended for infants.

Melissa *Melissa officinalis*

DESCRIPTION

Also known as lemon balm essential oil, Melissa essential oil is yellow in color and has a thin consistency. With a fresh, lemony scent, it may be used as a top or middle note in aromatherapy blends.

ORIGIN

Hungary, Italy, United States

PROPERTIES

Antibacterial, antihistaminic, anti-inflammatory, antiseptic, antispasmodic, antiviral, carminative, diaphoretic, digestive, febrifuge, sedative, tonic, uterine tonic, vermifuge

APPLICATION

Melissa essential oil may be used neat. It is suitable for direct inhalation, diffusion, topical application, and ingestion.

PRIMARY USES

Repels insects; calms coughs; soothes colds; lowers fevers; eases indigestion, menstrual pain, nausea, and stomach cramps; aids sedation and sleep.

When used for aromatherapy and in meditation, Melissa essential oil has a calming, uplifting effect. It helps ease emotional pressure, relieve tension, and restore balance and good spirits.

BLENDS WITH

Bergamot, citrus, chamomile, clary sage, frankincense, geranium, German chamomile, lavender, neroli, petitgrain, Roman chamomile, rose otto, yarrow

SAFE USE

Melissa essential oil is generally considered safe. It may cause skin irritation in some individuals.

Myrrh *Commiphora myrrha*

··

DESCRIPTION

Myrrh essential oil has a golden-yellow to brown color and a medium consistency. It is considered a base when used in aromatherapy blends, and its warm, earthy fragrance has woody undertones that give it an irresistible quality.

ORIGIN

Somalia

PROPERTIES

Antifungal, anti-inflammatory, antimicrobial, antiseptic, antispasmodic, antiviral, astringent, carminative, cicatrizant, emmenagogue, expectorant, sedative, tonic, vulnerary

APPLICATION

Myrrh essential oil may be used neat. It is suitable for direct inhalation, diffusion, topical application, and ingestion.

PRIMARY USES

Soothes bronchitis and coughs; eases diarrhea and dysentery; treats ringworm and athlete's foot; relieves painful tooth and gum conditions as well as canker sores; alleviates pain and discomfort caused by skin conditions; reduces appearance of wrinkles and stretch marks.

When used in aromatherapy and for meditation, myrrh essential oil aids in the release of fear and negativity. It uplifts the mind, relieves anxiety, and soothes stress.

BLENDS WITH

Bergamot, chamomile, clove, cypress, eucalyptus, frankincense, geranium, German chamomile, grapefruit, jasmine, juniper, lavender, lemon, lemon tea tree, mandarin, neroli, orange, palmarosa, patchouli, Roman chamomile, rosemary, rose otto, sandalwood, Scots pine, spikenard, tangerine, tea tree, vetiver, ylang-ylang

SAFE USE

Myrrh is generally regarded as safe. The FDA has approved it as a flavoring agent and food additive.

Myrrh has been popular for millennia. The Egyptians used it during the mummification process, and various religions throughout the world used it in their ceremonies. It is valued in Ayurvedic and Chinese medicine practices. The Bible mentions myrrh as one of the gifts of the Magi, and as an important anointing oil.

Myrtle *Myrtus communis*

....

DESCRIPTION

Myrtle essential oil is pale yellow in color and has a thin consistency. It has a sweet scent with floral and camphor undertones, and is useful as a top or middle note in aromatherapy blends.

ORIGIN

France, Spain, Tunisia

PROPERTIES

Antibacterial, antiseptic, astringent, expectorant, sedative, tonic

APPLICATION

Dilute myrtle essential oil 50:50 with a carrier oil. It may be diffused, directly inhaled, applied topically, or ingested.

PRIMARY USES

Improves oily skin and hair; treats minor skin infections; eases coughs and congestion; relieves insomnia.

When used for aromatherapy or in meditation, myrtle essential oil aids in releasing conflict and anger. It alleviates feelings of confusion and can help promote a sense of clarity.

BLENDS WITH

Bergamot, black pepper, clary sage, clove, ginger, hyssop, laurel, lavender, lemon, lime, rosemary

SAFE USE

Myrtle essential oil is generally regarded as safe. It is recognized by the FDA as both a food additive and a flavoring agent.

Neroli *Citrus aurantium*

··

DESCRIPTION

Neroli essential oil has a dark brown color and an intensely exotic floral aroma. It has a medium consistency and is used as a middle note in aromatherapy blends.

ORIGIN

France, Italy, Morocco, United States

PROPERTIES

Antibacterial, antifungal, anti-inflammatory, antiseptic, antispasmodic, aphrodisiac, carminative, sedative, tonic

APPLICATION

Dilute neroli essential oil 50:50 with a carrier oil. It may be directly inhaled, diffused, applied topically, or ingested.

PRIMARY USES

Eases cold symptoms; alleviates headaches; improves circulation; calms the nerves; aids oily and dry skin; reduces appearance of wrinkles and stretch marks.

When used in aromatherapy and for meditation, neroli essential oil helps alleviate anxiety and depression. It provides a grounding influence and aids in the release of pent-up emotions and the renewal of self-confidence.

BLENDS WITH

Allspice, benzoin, bergamot, cardamom, chamomile, clary sage, coriander, frankincense, geranium, German chamomile, ginger, grapefruit, Helichrysum, jasmine, juniper, lavender, lemon, lime, mandarin, myrrh, orange, palma-rosa, palo santo, patchouli, peppermint, petitgrain, Roman chamomile, rose otto, sandalwood, spikenard, tangerine, yarrow, ylang-ylang

SAFE USE

Neroli essential oil is generally considered safe for children, dogs, and horses.

Nutmeg *Myristica fragrans*

DESCRIPTION

Nutmeg essential oil is clear, with a thin consistency. It has a wonderfully rich, spicy fragrance and is used as a middle note in aromatherapy blends.

ORIGIN

Indonesia, Sri Lanka

PROPERTIES

Analgesic, antioxidant, antiseptic, antispasmodic, aphrodisiac, carminative, laxative, stimulant, tonic

APPLICATION

Dilute nutmeg essential oil 50:50 with a carrier oil. It is suitable for direct inhalation, diffusion, topical application, and ingestion.

PRIMARY USES

Eliminates halitosis and flatulence; soothes muscle aches and pains; increases circulation; relieves indigestion and diarrhea; improves appetite.

Historically, nutmeg essential oil was used to alleviate pain from ulcers and gallstones, and to support the adrenal glands. When used in aromatherapy or for meditation, nutmeg essential oil encourages spontaneity while releasing doubt, depression, and resistance to change.

BLENDS WITH

Bay, bergamot, carrot seed, chamomile, clary sage, coriander, geranium, German chamomile, lavender, lemon tea tree, lime, mandarin, oakmoss, orange, Peru balsam, petitgrain, Roman chamomile, rosemary, tangerine, tea tree

Nutmeg essential oil is generally regarded as safe and has been approved as a food additive by the FDA.

Many of nutmeg's medicinal uses are believed to have originated with the Chinese; today, nutmeg remains an important component in Chinese medicine. It is also contained in Hildegard von Bingen's medicine book, Physica, *which describes more than twelve thousand remedies for a variety of symptoms. Hildegard von Bingen was born in 1098, and was the first of the herbalists and naturopaths of the Middle Ages.*

Oakmoss *Evernia prunastri*

....

DESCRIPTION

Oakmoss essential oil is light brown in color, with a medium to thick consistency. It has a rich, earthy fragrance and is useful as a base in aromatherapy blends.

ORIGIN

France, United States

PROPERTIES

Antiseptic, demulcent, fixative

APPLICATION

Oakmoss essential oil must be heavily diluted. It may be diffused, directly inhaled, or applied topically. It is primarily useful in aromatherapy blends and is not suitable for ingestion.

PRIMARY USES

Soothes stiff joints and muscles; relieves coughs; alleviates cold symptoms.

When used in aromatherapy and for meditation, oakmoss essential oil typically enhances the effects of complementary oils. It is particularly useful for creating relaxing blends and for soothing inner turmoil.

BLENDS WITH

Angelica root, bay, bergamot, chamomile, clary sage, eucalyptus, galbanum, German chamomile, ginger, helichrysum, holy basil, juniper, lavender, lemon, lemon tea tree, lime, nutmeg, orange, palmarosa, patchouli, petitgrain, Roman chamomile, sandalwood, spikenard, spruce, star anise, tea tree, valerian, vetiver, yarrow, ylang-ylang

SAFE USE

Oakmoss essential oil can cause skin irritation. Do not apply to skin undiluted.

Orange *Citrus sinensis*

....

DESCRIPTION

Orange essential oil has two fragrances—sweet, which aptly has a sweet citrus fragrance, and bitter, which is much less popular and has a sharper aroma. If you have children and want to diffuse an essential oil in your home, this is a good choice. Greenish orange in color and with a thin consistency, this essential oil is typically expressed or cold pressed. When used in aromatherapy, it is considered a top note.

ORIGIN

Brazil, Italy, United States

PROPERTIES

Antidepressant, antiseptic, antispasmodic, antitumoral, circulatory, digestive, sedative, tonic

APPLICATION

Orange essential oil should be diluted 50:50 with a carrier oil prior to use. It is suitable for direct inhalation, diffusion, topical application, and ingestion.

PRIMARY USES

Soothes nervous tension and anxiety; combats depression; relieves insomnia and symptoms of menopause; improves skin tone; reduces appearance of wrinkles; improves digestion; eases hypertension, dyspepsia, and water retention.

Orange essential oil is a fragrant addition to nontoxic household products, lotions, massage oils, and bath products. It also has a calming effect on nervous dogs and skittish horses.

Orange essential oil can be used to promote a positive attitude as well as to calm the mind and ease feelings of aggravation. This wonderful essential oil can help you relax and stay focused while concentrating on tough mental tasks. When used for meditation, it promotes balance and aids in creativity while eliminating obsessiveness and fearfulness.

BLENDS WITH

Allspice, angelica root, basil, bergamot, black pepper, cardamom, catnip, cinnamon, clary sage, clove, coriander, eucalyptus, fir needle, frankincense, geranium, ginger, grapefruit, hyssop, jasmine, juniper, lavender, lemon, lemongrass, lemon tea tree, marjoram, myrrh, neroli, nutmeg, oakmoss, palmarosa, palo santo, patchouli, petitgrain, rose otto, sandalwood, spearmint, tea tree, vetiver, ylang-ylang

SAFE USE

Conduct a patch test before using orange essential oil on your skin. Dilute it by adding one part essential oil to one part carrier oil before topical use. Orange essential oil is slightly phototoxic, so avoid direct exposure to sunlight for twelve hours after use. Orange essential oil is also suitable for ingestion. To enjoy its many benefits, simply mix one or two drops into a glass of fresh water or herbal tea. Purchase only therapeutic-grade orange essential oil, particularly if you plan to ingest it or use it topically.

Do not expose cats to orange oil. They are naturally repulsed by it and will generally avoid it; however, you will need to contact your veterinarian if a cat swallows this essential oil.

Oranges have played an important role in Asian medicine since 2500 BCE. They are traditionally used to stimulate digestion, to relieve spasms, and even to bring good luck.

Palmarosa *Cymbopogon martinii*

DESCRIPTION

Palmarosa essential oil has a thin consistency and is pale yellow in color. It has a fresh, sweet, floral fragrance and is used as a middle note in aromatherapy compounds.

ORIGIN

Brazil, India

PROPERTIES

Antibacterial, antifungal, antiseptic, antiviral, digestive, febrifuge, stimulant, tonic

APPLICATION

Dilute palmarosa essential oil 50:50 with a carrier oil. It is suitable for direct inhalation, diffusion, topical application, and ingestion.

PRIMARY USES

Soothes digestive complaints; relieves stress and fatigue; softens scar tissue and dry skin; reduces appearance of wrinkles; soothes dermatitis; repels insects.

When used in aromatherapy or for meditation, palmarosa essential oil helps alleviate tension, promote inner clarity, and eliminate resentment.

BLENDS WITH

Bergamot, cardamom, cedar, chamomile, clary sage, clove, coriander, frankincense, geranium, German chamomile, ginger, grapefruit, helichrysum, jasmine, juniper, lavender, lemon, lemongrass, mandarin, myrrh, neroli, oakmoss, orange, palo santo, patchouli, petitgrain, Roman chamomile, rosemary, rose otto, sandalwood, spikenard, tangerine, ylang-ylang

Palmarosa is generally regarded as safe. Consume only therapeutic-grade palmarosa essential oil.

Palmarosa was used as incense by the ancient Egyptians, and in India it is often added to food to kill bacteria and promote healthy digestion.

Palo Santo *Bursera graveolens*

....

DESCRIPTION

Palo santo essential oil is clear to pale yellow in color and has a thin consistency. It has a sweet, woody aroma with hints of citrus and mint, and is used as a middle note in aromatherapy blends.

ORIGIN

Peru

PROPERTIES

Anti-infectious, anti-inflammatory, antiseptic, antiviral, immune-stimulant, sedative

APPLICATION

Dilute palo santo essential oil 50:50 with a carrier oil. It is suitable for direct inhalation, diffusion, and topical application.

PRIMARY USES

Stimulates the immune system; alleviates arthritis and rheumatism pain; relieves muscle pain and inflammation; repels insects; kills ticks.

When used in aromatherapy and for meditation, palo santo essential oil aids in releasing negative emotions, including anger and fear. It increases focus and alleviates confusion.

BLENDS WITH

Bergamot, black pepper, camphor, cinnamon, cypress, geranium, grapefruit, lavender, lemon, mandarin, neroli, orange, palmarosa, patchouli, rose otto, sandalwood, Scots pine, vetiver, wintergreen, ylang-ylang

Palo santo essential oil should not be ingested. It can cause skin irritation in some individuals if used neat; others use it without diluting and have no problems. Conduct a patch test before use.

Patchouli *Pogostemon cablin*

....

DESCRIPTION

Patchouli essential oil has a deep golden-brown color and a medium to thick consistency. Its rich, woody aroma is wonderfully appealing, and it makes an excellent base note in aromatherapy blends.

ORIGIN

India, Indonesia, Sri Lanka

PROPERTIES

Antibacterial, antiemetic, anti-inflammatory, antimicrobial, antiseptic, antiviral, carminative, decongestant, deodorant, febrifuge, laxative, stimulant, stomachic, tonic

APPLICATION

Patchouli essential oil may be used neat. It is suitable for direct inhalation, diffusion, topical application, and ingestion.

PRIMARY USES

Eases indigestion; alleviates constipation; soothes insect bites and stings, burns, and minor wounds; alleviates dandruff; moisturizes dry skin; reduces appearance of wrinkles; opens pores for cleansing; relieves oily skin and hair; repels insects.

When used in aromatherapy or for meditation, patchouli essential oil alleviates nervous exhaustion and relieves stress. It promotes physical and mental relaxation, increases focus, and helps users eliminate feelings of insecurity.

BLENDS WITH

Allspice, angelica root, bergamot, cardamom, chamomile, cinnamon, clary sage, clove, coriander, frankincense, geranium, German chamomile, ginger, grapefruit, jasmine, lavender, lemongrass, mandarin, myrrh, neroli, oakmoss, orange, palmarosa, palo santo, Peru balsam, petitgrain, Roman chamomile, rose otto, sandalwood, spikenard, tangerine, valerian, vetiver, ylang-ylang

SAFE USE

Patchouli essential oil is generally considered safe for humans, dogs, and horses. It is recognized as a flavoring agent and food additive by the FDA.

Patchouli thrives in tropical regions, but it is gaining increasing popularity as a houseplant in areas where outdoor temperatures are too cold for the plant to survive. If you live in a warm, humid region, you may enjoy growing patchouli outdoors. The plant prefers plenty of shade and a little indirect sunlight. Dried patchouli leaves make a great alternative to toxic mothballs.

Peppermint *Mentha piperita*

DESCRIPTION

Peppermint essential oil is an amazing medicinal with a very strong aroma. It is widely used in a number of commercially produced products, and it makes a fantastic addition to many aromatherapy blends. Peppermint essential oil is derived from the leaves of *Mentha piperita.* This plant is prolific and easy to cultivate, making peppermint essential oil one of the least expensive on the market. This essential oil has a thin consistency and is typically steam distilled. In aromatherapy, it is used as a top note.

ORIGIN

Egypt, Hungary, United States

PROPERTIES

Analgesic, antibacterial, anticarcinogenic, anti-inflammatory, antiparasitic, antispasmodic, antitumoral, antiviral, digestive

APPLICATION

Peppermint essential oil should be diluted 50:50 with a carrier oil prior to use. It is suitable for direct inhalation, diffusion, topical application, and ingestion.

PRIMARY USES

Soothes aches, pains, and itchy skin, including psoriasis and eczema; eases tension and headaches; soothes respiratory infections and asthma; relieves nausea and other digestive problems; combats viral and fungal infections, including cold sores.

Peppermint essential oil provides a wonderful cooling sensation due to the high level of menthol it contains, and when used in a body mist, it provides a fast cooldown. It makes an excellent liniment for relaxing horses' muscles, and when horses inhale it prior to a training session, they often focus better. Peppermint essential oil is useful in the creation of nontoxic household products. It is also an aphrodisiac, particularly when diffused. When used in aromatherapy, peppermint essential oil promotes greater mental focus and can help make learning new information easier. It is useful for calming the mind and easing fear. In meditation, this essential oil helps break down resistance concerning new situations; it is also useful for increasing intuitive awareness.

BLENDS WITH

Basil, benzoin, black pepper, catnip, cypress, eucalyptus, geranium, grapefruit, juniper, lavender, lemon, lemon tea tree, marjoram, niaouli, Ravensara, rosemary, Scots pine, spearmint, tea tree, wintergreen

SAFE USE

Conduct a patch test before using peppermint essential oil on your skin. It must be diluted prior to application; blend one part peppermint oil with one part carrier oil before using it in products that will come into contact with your skin. If you get peppermint oil in your eyes or on a cut, expect to feel a severe stinging sensation. Do not apply water, as this will only make the feeling intensify. Flushing the area with a carrier oil will provide relief. Children younger than six years old do not tolerate peppermint essential oil well. Anyone with high blood pressure should avoid contact or ingestion.

Peppermint essential oil is a fantastic tonic when taken internally. Blend a single drop with a glass of water or a cup of herbal tea for a refreshing beverage. Ingest therapeutic-grade peppermint essential oil to receive health benefits; food-grade oil is not the same.

The genus name for peppermint, Mentha, *comes from a Greek myth in which the nymph Mentha is pursued by the god Pluto. His jealous wife, Persephone, crushes Mentha to dust. Pluto resurrects Mentha as a sweetly aromatic peppermint plant that is notoriously difficult to eradicate.*

Peru Balsam *Myroxylon balsamum*

DESCRIPTION

Peru balsam essential oil has a soft, fresh, earthy aroma most people love. It is dark brown with a thick consistency and is suitable for use as a base note in aromatherapy blends.

ORIGIN

Central America, France

PROPERTIES

Anti-inflammatory, antiseptic, expectorant, stimulant

APPLICATION

Peru balsam essential oil is so thick that it's almost a resin. It may be applied topically, but heavy dilution is recommended as some individuals are extremely sensitive to it. It is most useful for aromatherapy; it can be diffused after dilution or inhaled directly.

PRIMARY USES

Alleviates coughs and other cold symptoms; soothes rashes and minor wounds.

Peru balsam essential oil is excellent for use as a scent fixative and base note in body care products. When used in aromatherapy and for meditation, Peru balsam essential oil promotes relaxation and soothes the senses.

BLENDS WITH

Black pepper, ginger, jasmine, lavender, nutmeg, patchouli, petitgrain, rose otto, sandalwood, ylang-ylang

SAFE USE

Women who are pregnant or breastfeeding should avoid Peru balsam essential oil. Do not ingest this essential oil.

Petitgrain *Citrus aurantium*

DESCRIPTION

Petitgrain essential oil is clear to pale yellow in color and has a thin consistency. It has a fresh, woody fragrance and is used as a top note in aromatherapy blends.

ORIGIN

France, North Africa

PROPERTIES

Antiseptic, antispasmodic, carminative, deodorant, stimulant, tonic

APPLICATION

Dilute petitgrain essential oil 50:50 with a carrier oil. It may be directly inhaled, diffused, applied topically, and ingested.

PRIMARY USES

Alleviates anxiety; soothes muscle and digestive spasms; alleviates excessive perspiration; aids sleep.

When used in aromatherapy and for meditation, petitgrain essential oil can help release avoidance and denial. It is an excellent aid for those attempting to overcome addictions and embrace self-worth.

BLENDS WITH

Bergamot, cardamom, cedarwood, clary sage, clove, cypress, eucalyptus lemon, frankincense, geranium, jasmine, juniper, lavender, lemon,, mandarin, marjoram, Melissa, neroli, nutmeg, oakmoss, orange, palmarosa, patchouli, Peru balsam, rosemary, rose otto, sandalwood, tangerine, valerian, ylang-ylang

SAFE USE

Petitgrain essential oil is generally considered safe.

Roman Chamomile *Anthemis nobilis*

DESCRIPTION

Roman chamomile is derived from the flowers of chamomile species *Anthemis nobilis*. With a sweet fragrance, at once fresh, soft, and herbaceous, with apple undertones that remind one of a sunny day in an apple orchard, Roman chamomile is a favorite essential oil with many uses. An effective essential oil for irritation and impatience, Roman chamomile offers relief from PMS, and other menstrual and menopausal issues. This essential oil has a thin consistency and is grayish to pale blue in color. When used in aromatherapy, it is a middle note. Although Roman chamomile can be used as an herbal tea, particularly for medicinal purposes, it is German chamomile that is more often found in beverages. Roman and German chamomile are two different species, although they are closely related and both possess calming properties.

ORIGIN

France, Hungary, Italy, United States

PROPERTIES

Analgesic, antibiotic, anti-inflammatory, antimicrobial, antineuritic, antiseptic, antispasmodic, carminative, digestive, emmenagogue, febrifuge, hepatic, sedative, stomachic, sudorific, tonic, vermifuge, vulnerary

APPLICATION

Roman chamomile essential oil may be used neat. It is suitable for direct inhalation, diffusion, and topical application. It is also suitable for ingestion.

PRIMARY USES

Reduces pain from muscle aches, strains, sprains, minor wounds, headaches, and arthritic pain; calms irritated skin; soothes allergies, insect bites, and earaches; eases premenstrual symptoms; soothes frazzled nerves; reduces feelings of anger and irritability; promotes deep relaxation; relieves insomnia.

This essential oil is useful for formulating nontoxic household products, lotions, massage oils, bath products, and calming spray. It is safe for most animals and can help calm nervous pets.

Roman chamomile essential oil is famous for its use as an anti-inflammatory. It can also be used to promote a sense of calm and is one of the few essential oils appropriate for diffusing around young babies and cranky toddlers. When used for meditation, Roman chamomile essential oil promotes feelings of well-being and helps eliminate confusion, fear, and doubt.

BLENDS WITH

Angelica root, benzoin, bergamot, citrus, clary sage, clove, cypress, eucalyptus, frankincense, geranium, grapefruit, helichrysum, jasmine, lavender, lemon, lemon tea tree, marjoram, Melissa, mountain savory, myrrh, myrtle, neroli, nutmeg, oakmoss, palmarosa, patchouli, rosemary, rose otto, sandalwood, tea tree, yarrow, ylang-ylang

SAFE USE

Conduct a patch test before using Roman chamomile essential oil on your skin. This is one of the few essential oils considered safe to apply undiluted; however, despite its widespread use in commercially produced calming skin creams, some individuals can suffer skin irritation when the oil is applied topically.

Roman chamomile essential oil is safe for ingestion. A drop or two in a cup of herbal tea or water has an almost instantaneous calming effect, and also makes an excellent tonic for easing digestive gas and bloating. As Roman chamomile essential oil has a relaxing effect, it may increase drowsiness when used in conjunction with sedatives.

In ancient Egypt, chamomile was often used as an offering to Ra, the sun god. It was also used as a strewing herb—scattered on the floor of homes and other buildings—throughout history, and is famous for its ability to take the place of hops in brewing beer.

Rosemary *Rosmarinus officinalis*

....

DESCRIPTION

Rosemary essential oil is extremely versatile, as it is useful for treating a number of illnesses as well as for aromatherapy and meditation. It is derived from the flowers of *Rosmarinus officinalis.* Though some companies provide rosemary oil derived from other rosemary species with similar fragrances, those oils have different properties. Rosemary essential oil is an evergreen, but its fragrance is not overly woody. Instead, it is fresh, sweet, and strongly herbal, with slightly medicinal undertones. With a thin consistency, this essential oil is typically steam distilled. When used in aromatherapy, it is considered a middle note.

ORIGIN

France, Spain, Tunisia

PROPERTIES

Analgesic, antiarthritic, antibacterial, antifungal, antioxidant, antirheumatic, antiseptic, antispasmodic, aphrodisiac, astringent, carminative, cordial, decongestant, diaphoretic, digestive, diuretic, emmenagogue, expectorant, hepatic, hypertensive, nervine, restorative, rubefacient, stimulant, stomachic, sudorific, tonic, vermifuge, vulnerary

APPLICATION

Rosemary essential oil should be diluted 50:50 with a carrier oil prior to use. It is suitable for direct inhalation, diffusion, and topical application. It is also suitable for ingestion.

PRIMARY USES

Improves circulation; eases arthritis and rheumatism pain; relieves muscle cramps; combats dandruff, hair loss, and dull skin; reduces oily skin and acne; alleviates respiratory discomfort; helps colds and congestion; repels insects.

Rosemary essential oil can be used to formulate nontoxic disinfectants and other household products, bath products, and lotions. It is an excellent addition to massage oils, particularly when blended with lavender. It is extremely stimulating to the mind and is great for combating mental fatigue. Heralded for its ability to help users remain focused and alert while studying, working on mentally draining projects, and driving long distances, rosemary essential oil is even a great natural remedy for easing mental fog caused by hangovers.

When used in meditation, rosemary essential oil alleviates stress and anxiety, aids in promoting focus and mental clarity, and increases intuition.

BLENDS WITH

Basil, bergamot, black pepper, blue cypress, catnip, cedarwood, chamomile, cinnamon, citronella, clary sage, Douglas fir, elemi, eucalyptus, fir needle, frankincense, geranium, German chamomile, grapefruit, helichrysum, hyssop, juniper, lavender, lemon, lemongrass, lemon tea tree, *Litsea cubeba*, mandarin, marjoram, myrrh, myrtle, niaouli, nutmeg, oregano, palmarosa, peppermint, petitgrain, Ravensara, Roman chamomile, sage, Scots pine, spearmint, spruce, tea tree, thyme, valerian.

SAFE USE

Conduct a patch test before using rosemary essential oil on your skin. This is one of the few essential oils that is considered to be safe for applying undiluted; however, some individuals can suffer skin irritation when the oil is applied topically. Rosemary essential oil can be toxic if ingested, and is best for aromatherapy and topical applications.

Rosemary is considered a harbinger of wealth. When placed near the entrance to a home or business, it is said to increase income. It is also a symbol of love—rosemary sprigs tied with colorful ribbons were often presented to wedding guests in days past.

Rose Otto *Rosa damascena*

....

DESCRIPTION

Rose otto essential oil is light yellow in color and has a thin consistency. It is much less costly than thick, dark red rose absolute, and it provides the same benefits. When used in aromatherapy blends, it is considered a middle note.

ORIGIN

Bulgaria, France, Turkey

PROPERTIES

Analgesic, antibacterial, antifungal, antimicrobial, antiseptic, antiviral, aphrodisiac, astringent, deodorant, disinfectant, diuretic, hepatic, sedative, stomachic, tonic

APPLICATION

Rose otto essential oil may be used neat. It is suitable for direct inhalation, diffusion, topical application, and ingestion.

PRIMARY USES

Soothes minor burns, cuts, and abrasions; relieves dry, chapped skin; reduces appearance of wrinkles; alleviates headaches, including migraines.

When used in aromatherapy or for meditation, rose otto essential oil can help improve memory and concentration. It is excellent for relieving stress and alleviating nervous tension.

BLENDS WITH

Bergamot, black pepper, chamomile, cinnamon, clary sage, clove, cypress, fennel, frankincense, geranium, German chamomile, ginger, helichrysum, holy basil, jasmine, lavender, lemon, mandarin, Melissa, myrrh, neroli, orange, palmarosa, palo santo, patchouli, Peru balsam, petitgrain, Roman chamomile, sandalwood, spikenard, tangerine, vetiver, ylang-ylang

Rose otto essential oil is generally recognized as safe. Select only therapeutic-grade essential oil as there are many shoddy substitutes on the market.

Fossil records show that roses have grown on our planet for approximately thirty-five million years—in a fascinating array of shapes, colors, and sizes. Some can live for centuries. The oldest living rose grows on a wall at Hildesheim, in Germany. Its presence has been documented there ever since 815 CE.

Sage *Salvia officinalis*

....

DESCRIPTION

Also called "common sage," sage essential oil has a thin consistency and a fresh, herbaceous scent. With a strong camphor characteristic and a hint of fruit, this essential oil is considered a top note when used in aromatherapy blends.

ORIGIN

Spain, Ukraine, United States

PROPERTIES

Antibacterial, anti-inflammatory, antimicrobial, antioxidant, antiseptic, antispasmodic, astringent, digestive, diuretic, febrifuge, insecticide, laxative, stomachic, tonic

APPLICATION

Inhale directly or diffuse sage essential oil, and dilute it prior to topical application.

PRIMARY USES

Repels insects; soothes skin; reduces appearance of scars; alleviates dandruff; reduces premenstrual symptoms; stimulates bile production; eases coughs; promotes healthy metabolism.

The antibacterial and antimicrobial properties of sage essential oil makes it great for use in household cleaners.

BLENDS WITH

Chamomile, citrus, German chamomile, hyssop, juniper, lavender, lemon, Roman chamomile, rosemary, rosewood, Scots pine

Sage essential oil has an extremely high thujone concentration and can cause severe skin irritation when applied neat. Those with sensitive skin should avoid using it altogether. Women who are pregnant should avoid contact with sage, as should people with epilepsy. Sage essential oil is not suitable for ingestion.

Sandalwood *Santalum album*

....

DESCRIPTION

Sandalwood essential oil boasts a number of health benefits and is excellent for use in natural cleaning products. There are many different sandalwood species that have been shown to have little to no medicinal value, so be certain you purchase only *Santalum album* essential oil. With a medium to thick consistency, this essential oil is typically steam distilled, and when used in aromatherapy, it is considered a base note.

ORIGIN

Australia

PROPERTIES

Antidepressant, antiseptic, antitumoral, antiviral, aphrodisiac, astringent, bronchial dilator, calming, immune stimulant, sedative, tonic

APPLICATION

Sandalwood essential oil may be used neat. It is suitable for direct inhalation, diffusion, topical application, and ingestion.

PRIMARY USES

Reduces wrinkles, scars, and acne; combats viral infections, including cold sores; treats urinary tract infections; combats inflammations, including bronchitis; eases diarrhea; soothes hemorrhoids; aids sleep.

Sandalwood essential oil can be used to formulate nontoxic household products, bath products, lotions, shampoos, and conditioners. It is useful for calming and relaxing stressed or anxious dogs, horses, and humans, and in people it is known to promote a sense of calm and inner peace as well as to ease feelings of mental cloudiness. When used for meditation, it promotes intuition; it even helps users to let go of painful old memories and emotional issues.

Benzoin, bergamot, black pepper, blue cypress, cardamom, chamomile, citronella, clary sage, clove, fennel, frankincense, geranium, German chamomile, ginger, grapefruit, jasmine, lavender, lemon, mandarin, myrrh, neroli, oakmoss, orange, palmarosa, palo santo, patchouli, Peru balsam, petitgrain, Roman chamomile, rose otto, rosewood, Scots pine, tangerine, tuberose, vetiver, ylang-ylang

SAFE USE

Though safe and generally non-irritating, sandalwood essential oil should be diluted prior to use. Add one part sandalwood oil to one part carrier oil for topical use, and conduct a patch test before using it on your skin. Sandalwood essential oil may be taken internally. Ingest only one drop at a time, ensuring you mix it carefully with water or herbal tea. As sandalwood essential oil has a relaxing effect, it may increase drowsiness when used in conjunction with sedatives.

As many as four thousand years ago, sandalwood was used as an aid to meditation in religious ceremonies throughout Egypt, Greece, India, and Rome. The wood was also used to build temples, and Egyptians used sandalwood essential oil in embalming recipes.

Scots Pine   *Pinus sylvestris*

....

DESCRIPTION

Although derived from *Pinus sylvestris,* or Scots pine, manufacturers often use a shortened label, such as "pine" or "pine needle" for this essential oil. Clear, with a medium, slightly oily consistency, Scots pine essential oil has a wonderfully fragrant aroma and is used as a middle note in aromatherapy blends.

ORIGIN

Bulgaria, Hungary, United States

PROPERTIES

Analgesic, antibacterial, antifungal, anti-inflammatory, antimicrobial, antineuritic, antiseptic, antiviral, balsamic, decongestant, deodorant, disinfectant, diuretic, insecticide, vermifuge

APPLICATION

Dilute Scots pine essential oil 50:50 with a carrier oil. It is suitable for direct inhalation, diffusion, topical application, and ingestion.

PRIMARY USES

Soothes coughs and other cold symptoms; alleviates muscle aches and pains; improves circulation; eliminates fluid retention.

Scots pine essential oil is excellent for use in nontoxic household cleansers. When used in aromatherapy or for meditation, Scots pine essential oil promotes feelings of peace and relaxation. It helps alleviate nervous tension and release stress while promoting an overall sense of well-being.

Bergamot, cedarwood, citronella, clary sage, cypress, Douglas fir, eucalyptus, fir needle, frankincense, galbanum, grapefruit, juniper, lavender,
lemon, lemon tea tree, marjoram, myrrh, palo santo, peppermint, rosemary, sage, sandalwood, spearmint, spikenard, spruce, tea tree, thyme,
valerian, yarrow

SAFE USE

Scots pine essential oil may cause skin irritation in some individuals.

Spearmint *Mentha spicata*

DESCRIPTION

Spearmint essential oil is clear, with a thin consistency. It has a minty aroma with fruity undertones and is used as a top note in formulating aromatherapy blends.

ORIGIN

Hungary, Nepal, United States

PROPERTIES

Analgesic, anesthetic, antibacterial, anti-inflammatory, antiseptic, antispasmodic, astringent, cephalic, decongestant, digestive, diuretic, expectorant, febrifuge, hepatic, stimulant, tonic

APPLICATION

Dilute one part spearmint essential oil with two parts carrier oil. Spearmint essential oil may be directly inhaled, diffused, applied topically, and ingested.

PRIMARY USES

Relieves cold and flu symptoms, including cough and congestion; alleviates headaches, nausea, vomiting, and flatulence; stimulates metabolism.

Spearmint essential oil can be used in place of peppermint essential oil; it has a milder fragrance and similar effects. When used in aromatherapy or for meditation, spearmint essential oil promotes relaxation and relieves feelings of stress and nervous tension. It also aids in promoting an overall sense of balance and well-being.

Basil, catnip, chamomile, eucalyptus, German chamomile, jasmine, lavender, lemon, orange, peppermint, Roman chamomile, rosemary

SAFE USE

Spearmint essential oil is generally regarded as safe. Dilute prior to topical application to prevent skin irritation.

Spikenard *Nardostachys jatamansi*

....

DESCRIPTION

Spikenard essential oil has a deep golden-yellow color and a medium consistency. Its woody, earthy fragrance makes it ideal for use as a base note in aromatherapy blends.

ORIGIN

Nepal, United States

PROPERTIES

Antibacterial, antibiotic, antifungal, anti-infectious, anti-inflammatory, antiseptic, deodorant, laxative, sedative, tonic

APPLICATION

Spikenard essential oil may be used neat. It is suitable for direct inhalation, diffusion, topical application, and ingestion.

PRIMARY USES

Alleviates rashes and mild bacterial infections, including athlete's foot; relieves menstrual cramps and premenstrual symptoms; soothes inflamed skin; softens appearance of wrinkles; aids sleep.

When used in aromatherapy or for meditation, spikenard essential oil helps release tension and alleviate stress.

BLENDS WITH

Cistus, clary sage, clove, cypress, frankincense, geranium, juniper, lavender, lemon, myrrh, neroli, oakmoss, palmarosa, patchouli, rose otto, Scots pine, vetiver

Spikenard essential oil is generally regarded as safe.

Spikenard was a valuable essential oil in ancient times, just as it is today. Spikenard oil and ointment were stored in precious alabaster boxes with tight-fitting lids to keep air and light out.

Spruce *Tsuga canadensis*

....

DESCRIPTION

Spruce essential oil is clear, with a thin consistency and a fresh, woody aroma. It is used as a middle note in compounding aromatherapy blends.

ORIGIN

Canada, United States

PROPERTIES

Antimicrobial, antiseptic, astringent, diaphoretic, diuretic, expectorant, nervine, rubefacient, tonic

APPLICATION

Dilute spruce essential oil 50:50 with a carrier oil. It may be inhaled directly, diffused, applied topically, and ingested.

PRIMARY USES

Alleviates muscle aches and pains; relieves colds and coughs; increases circulation.

Spruce essential oil is excellent for use in nontoxic household cleaners. When used in aromatherapy or for meditation, spruce essential oil has a balancing, grounding effect. It releases emotional blocks to wealth and prosperity while promoting feelings of stability.

BLENDS WITH

Cedar, chamomile, clary sage, galbanum, German chamomile, lavender, oakmoss, Roman chamomile, rosemary, Scots pine

SAFE USE

Spruce essential oil is generally regarded as safe. Applying without first diluting can cause skin irritation in some individuals.

Tangerine *Citrus reticulata*

....

DESCRIPTION

Tangerine essential oil is greenish orange in color, with a thin consistency. It has a fresh, sweet citrus fragrance and is used as a top note in aromatherapy blends.

ORIGIN

China, United States

PROPERTIES

Antimicrobial, antiseptic, antispasmodic, carminative, digestive, diuretic, hypnotic, laxative, stimulant, tonic

APPLICATION

Dilute tangerine essential oil 50:50 with a carrier oil. It may be directly inhaled, diffused, applied topically, and ingested.

PRIMARY USES

Increases circulation; eliminates water retention; decongests lymphatic system; promotes healthy metabolism.

When used in aromatherapy or for meditation, tangerine essential oil has a calming, centering effect. It is helpful in promoting awareness, particularly in individuals who are working toward realizing goals.

BLENDS WITH

Angelica root, basil, black pepper, cinnamon, clary sage, clove, fir needle, frankincense, geranium, grapefruit, jasmine, juniper, lemon, myrrh, neroli, nutmeg, palmarosa, patchouli, petitgrain, rose otto, sandalwood, ylang-ylang

SAFE USE

Tangerine essential oil is sometimes phototoxic; avoid exposure to direct sunlight for at least twenty-four hours after use. It is toxic to cats.

Tea Tree *Melaleuca alternifolia*

....

DESCRIPTION

Tea tree essential oil is a pale yellow oil, with a thin consistency and a fresh, herbaceous medicinal aroma. When used in aromatherapy blends, it is considered a middle note.

ORIGIN

Australia, New South Wales

PROPERTIES

Antibacterial, antifungal, antimicrobial, antiseptic, antiviral, balsamic, expectorant, insecticide, stimulant, sudorific

APPLICATION

Dilute tea tree oil 50:50 with a carrier oil before diffusing or applying to skin. It may be used as a digestive supplement, and it is suitable for direct inhalation.

PRIMARY USES

Relieves colds, sinusitis, and bronchitis; stimulates the immune system; clears acne; alleviates skin irritation.

BLENDS WITH

Chamomile, cinnamon, clary sage, clove, echinacea, geranium, German chamomile, helichrysum, lavender, lemon, lemongrass, myrrh, nutmeg, oakmoss, peppermint, Roman chamomile, rosemary, rosewood, Scots pine, thyme

SAFE USE

Tea tree essential oil is generally regarded as safe. Always dilute prior to applying to skin, as it can cause irritation. Contact sensitization can occur if used repeatedly.

Valerian *Valeriana officinalis*

....

DESCRIPTION

Valerian essential oil has a warm, woody fragrance with musky undertones.
It is used as a base in aromatherapy blends.

ORIGIN

China, France, Hungary

PROPERTIES

Antibacterial, antispasmodic, carminative, diuretic, hypnotic, hypotensive,
sedative, stomachic

APPLICATION

Valerian essential oil may be used neat. It is suitable for direct inhalation,
diffusion, topical application, and ingestion.

PRIMARY USES

Aids sedation and sleep; soothes restless leg syndrome, menstrual cramps,
tension headaches, and tendinitis; alleviates hyperactivity.

When used in aromatherapy or for meditation, valerian essential oil
calms and relaxes overworked minds while alleviating stress and
promoting balance.

BLENDS WITH

Cedarwood, lavender, mandarin, oakmoss, patchouli, petitgrain, rosemary,
Scots pine, yarrow

Valerian essential oil may cause skin irritation. Avoid large doses, and do not take it for an extended period of time.

Historically, valerian was a popular ingredient for compounding love potions and aphrodisiacs.

Vetiver *Vetiveria zizanioides*

....

DESCRIPTION

Vetiver essential oil is a dark golden-brown color and has a thick consistency. It has a spicy, woody aroma and is used as a base note in aromatherapy blends.

ORIGIN

Haiti, Indonesia, Sri Lanka

PROPERTIES

Analgesic, antibacterial, antifungal, anti-inflammatory, antimicrobial, antioxidant, antiseptic, antispasmodic, cell proliferant, depurative, emmenagogue, rubefacient, sedative, stimulant, tonic, vermifuge, vulnerary

APPLICATION

Vetiver essential oil may be applied neat; however, it is thick and may be easier to use if diluted 50:50 in a carrier oil. It is suitable for direct inhalation, diffusion, topical application, and ingestion.

PRIMARY USES

Soothes acne, vitiligo, and dry skin; rejuvenates aching muscles and sore feet; alleviates pain caused by tendinitis, joint stiffness, menstrual cramps, and muscular dystrophy; reduces attention deficit hyperactivity disorder (ADHD) symptoms.

When used in aromatherapy or for meditation, vetiver essential oil can combat absentmindedness, alleviate depression, and provide an overall sense of calm.

Angelica root, bergamot, black pepper, cardamom, cedarwood, clary sage, frankincense, geranium, ginger, grapefruit, helichrysum, jasmine, lavender, lemon, lemongrass, *Litsea cubeba,* mandarin, myrrh, oakmoss, opopanax, orange, palo santo, patchouli, rose otto, sandalwood, spikenard, wintergreen, yarrow, ylang-ylang.

SAFE USE

Vetiver is generally regarded as safe.

Vetiver was commonly used in folk magic to increase abundance and facilitate communication with fairies, gnomes, and elves.

Wintergreen *Gaultheria procumbens*

....

DESCRIPTION

Wintergreen essential oil is clear, with a thin consistency. It has a strong fragrance and is useful as a top note in preparing aromatherapy blends.

ORIGIN

Canada, United States

PROPERTIES

Analgesic, anticoagulant, anti-inflammatory, antirheumatic, antiseptic, antispasmodic, disinfectant, stimulant, vasodilator

APPLICATION

Dilute one part essential oil in four parts carrier oil. Wintergreen essential oil is suitable for direct inhalation and diffusion.

PRIMARY USES

Relieves fibromyalgia, arthritis, and rheumatism pain; soothes cold and flu symptoms; alleviates muscle spasms, cramps, and irritable bowel symptom; tames headaches.

Wintergreen essential oil is useful in mouth rinses and in nontoxic household cleaners. When used in aromatherapy or for meditation, wintergreen essential oil promotes concentration and increases awareness.

BLENDS WITH

Balsam fir, clove, eucalyptus, helichrysum, juniper, lemon, lemongrass, marjoram, oregano, palo santo, peppermint, thyme, vetiver

SAFE USE

Wintergreen essential oil is very powerful and potentially hazardous. It can cause skin irritation if applied undiluted, and it should not be swallowed.

Pure, undiluted wintergreen oil is extremely poisonous to humans if taken internally, in as little as 10-milliliter doses. A teaspoon of pure wintergreen oil can be fatal to a child. Wintergreen contains high concentrations of methyl salicylate, the active ingredient of aspirin, and anyone with aspirin/salicylate sensitivities should avoid wintergreen completely.

Do not use wintergreen topically in large doses, do not use it undiluted, and do not use it for more than three days out of any month. Do not use on children, pets, or on pregnant women. Since the compounds are absorbed through the skin, wintergreen can be dangerous to anyone suffering from liver or kidney disease, or anyone taking blood thinners, such as warfarin. Use common sense in labeling anything containing wintergreen, keep out of reach of children, and be sure to triple-check for any allergies or sensitivities before use.

Yarrow *Achillea millefolium*

....

DESCRIPTION

Yarrow essential oil is yellow, green, or dark blue, with a medium consistency and a strong, herbaceous aroma with hints of wood. It is used as a middle note in aromatherapy blends.

ORIGIN

Bosnia, France, Hungary, United States

PROPERTIES

Antiarthritic, antibacterial, antifungal, anti-inflammatory, antiseptic, antispasmodic, astringent, carminative, diaphoretic, digestive, emmenagogue, expectorant, febrifuge, stimulant, tonic, vulnerary

APPLICATION

Apply yarrow essential oil neat for treating wounds; dilute it 50:50 with a carrier oil for other purposes. Yarrow essential oil may be applied topically, inhaled directly, diffused, and ingested.

PRIMARY USES

Relieves inflammation, including cold symptoms; soothes minor burns and wounds; helps cuts heal faster; reduces appearance of scars, stretch marks, and varicose veins; decreases hypertension; promotes hair growth; stimulates scalp.

When used in aromatherapy for meditation, yarrow essential oil helps promote feelings of tranquillity while easing tumultuous thoughts, feelings of irritation, and anger.

Bay, bergamot, black pepper, cedar, chamomile, clary sage, cypress, echinacea, grapefruit, German chamomile, lavender, Melissa, neroli, oakmoss, Roman chamomile, Scots pine, valerian, vetiver, ylang-ylang

SAFE USE

Yarrow essential oil is generally considered safe. Women who are pregnant should avoid contact, and some individuals suffer photosensitivity or rashes after use. Conduct a patch test prior to application, particularly if you have sensitive skin.

Ylang-Ylang   *Cananga odorata* or *C. odorata* var. *genuina*

DESCRIPTION

The most effective grade of ylang-ylang essential oil is Ylang-Ylang Complete or Ylang-Ylang I. Ylang-ylang essential oil is a sweet-smelling floral, and in Indonesia, it is called "poor man's jasmine." Though fragrant, its aroma is not overpowering. It is slightly fruity and delicate, with a fresh scent that is intensely appealing to most. With a medium consistency, this essential oil is typically steam distilled, and when used in aromatherapy, it may be used as a middle or base note.

ORIGIN

Comoro Islands, Madagascar

PROPERTIES

Antidepressant, antidiabetic, anti-inflammatory, antispasmodic, antiseptic, sedative, tonic, vasodilator

APPLICATION

Ylang-ylang essential oil may be used neat. It is suitable for direct inhalation, diffusion, topical application, and ingestion.

PRIMARY USES

Treats anxiety, depression, and insomnia; releases tension in mind and muscles; soothes irritated skin and appearance of wrinkles; stimulates new cell growth; relieves acne; eases intestinal discomfort; reduces hypertension; promotes smooth skin and thick hair.

Ylang-ylang essential oil has a calming effect on animals, including dogs, cats, and horses. It is also a fantastic addition to body care blends for the bath, and it is marvelous when blended into massage oil.

When used in aromatherapy, ylang-ylang essential oil helps release negative emotions, including low self-esteem, possessiveness, and anger, while promoting confidence, spiritual awareness, and self-acceptance. When used for meditation, it helps increase awareness and bring the body, mind, and spirit into greater alignment with one another. It is also an excellent oil to use if you are working to cultivate gratitude in your life.

BLENDS WITH

Allspice, bergamot, cardamom, chamomile, cinnamon, clary sage, clove, cypress, eucalyptus lemon, frankincense, geranium, German chamomile, ginger, grapefruit, helichrysum, jasmine, lemon, lemongrass, mandarin, myrrh, neroli, oakmoss, opopanax, orange, palmarosa, palo santo, patchouli, Peru balsam, petitgrain, Roman chamomile, rose otto, rosewood, sandalwood, tangerine, tuberose, vetiver, yarrow

SAFE USE

Conduct a patch test before using ylang-ylang essential oil on your skin. This is one of the few essential oils that is considered safe to apply undiluted; however, some individuals can suffer skin irritation when it is applied topically. Use ylang-ylang sparingly at first, as some individuals are quite sensitive to its fragrance. When used in excess, it can lead to nausea and headaches.

Ylang-ylang essential oil is safe to ingest; mix a single drop into filtered water or herbal tea, and let the aroma and relaxing sensation it brings take you away.

Ylang-ylang is known for its ability to increase libido, so it's not surprising that newlyweds in Indonesia enter their bridal suites to find their beds covered in ylang-ylang flowers.

CHAPTER FIVE

Essential Oils for Ailments

BABY CARE

Natural Baby Powder

....

Many commercially-produced baby powders contain artificial fragrances and talc, both of which can cause irritation of a baby's skin and lungs. As such, talc is no longer recommended by most pediatricians. This delightfully scented baby powder is safer for your baby and is also ideal for helping adults stay cool and dry. The marigold essential oil is perfect for soothing sensitive skin.

```
1 cup arrowroot powder
8 drops marigold essential oil
```

Blend the essential oil and arrowroot powder together in a glass bowl, blender, or food processor. Store in a sugar shaker for easy access.

Soothing Baby Oil

If you don't like the idea of using petroleum-based baby oil on an infant, this vitamin-rich baby oil makes an outstanding substitute. The lavender and chamomile essential oils soothe fussiness, while the marigold helps protect tender skin.

```
4 drops marigold essential oil
2 drops lavender essential oil
2 drops chamomile essential oil
1 cup organic apricot kernel oil
```

Blend all the essential oils, then add them to the apricot kernel oil. Mix well and store in a glass bottle away from heat and sunlight. Apply as needed to moisturize and protect your baby's skin. This blend is also fantastic for soothing massages that people of all ages will appreciate.

Natural Diaper Rash Remedy

If your baby is suffering a diaper rash and you don't like the idea of using a commercial preparation with chemical components, try this natural diaper rash remedy. The lavender and yarrow essential oils soothe the skin and help eliminate bacteria.

```
10 drops lavender essential oil
10 drops yarrow essential oil
1 pint warm water
```

Blend the essential oils. Add one drop of the blend to the warm water just before diaper changes. Use a soft cloth soaked in the mixture to cleanse your baby; afterwards, use a clean cotton ball to apply additional solution to the diaper area.

Use this blend to create a soothing protective oil, too. Add 1 drop of the blend to 4 teaspoons of sweet almond oil or jojoba oil. Apply a light layer of protective oil before diapering your baby.

Preventing the Flu

There's no need to worry next time the flu begins making its rounds. Conifer and eucalyptus essential oils have antiviral properties that can help keep flu germs from spreading.

```
1 drop fir needle essential oil
1 drop Scots pine essential oil
1 drop eucalyptus essential oil
3 drops carrier oil of choice
```

Blend all the oils together, add them to a diffuser, and use the mixture in your home or office throughout flu season. This blend may also be added to a spray bottle filled with 3 ounces of water. Use it to clean doorknobs and other items multiple people handle throughout the day.

Alleviating Flu-Related Joint Pain

Joint and muscle pain go hand in hand with influenza. Lavender oil helps soothe sore joints, and its gentle sedative property encourages relaxation.

```
10 drops lavender essential oil
1 ounce carrier oil of choice
```

Blend the oils together and gently massage the affected area. This blend is suitable for children as well as adults.

Sore Throat Spray

....

If you have a sore throat, this simple, natural spray will provide rapid relief. Peppermint and lemon essential oils have anti-inflammatory properties, and the lemon essential oil in this remedy provides a helpful vitamin C boost.

1/4 cup distilled water
1/4 cup fresh lemon juice
20 drops lemon essential oil
7 drops peppermint essential oil

Blend all the ingredients together in a spray bottle. Shake well before spritzing the mixture into the mouth, toward the rear of the throat. Use as needed. Keep in refrigerator for up to 2 weeks.

Sore Throat Gargle

....

A sore throat is often one of the first symptoms of a cold or flu. The echinacea essential oil this simple gargle contains helps soothe the pain while stimulating the body's immune system.

3 drops echinacea essential oil
3 ounces warm water

Blend the essential oil with the water, stirring vigorously. Immediately gargle, using small amounts until the entire mixture is gone. Repeat this treatment at least twice daily for best results.

Ginger Tea Relief

Tea is a traditional remedy for cold symptoms. When you add ginger essential oil to your favorite tea, you benefit additionally from its powerful antiviral compounds.

```
1 cup of hot herbal tea
1 drop ginger essential oil
```

Brew a tea of your choice. Once it's cool enough to drink, add the ginger essential oil to your cup. Inhaling the fragrance while sipping the tea provides relief from congestion; ingesting the ginger can help shorten your cold's duration. Drink this tea throughout the day for best results.

Herbal Steam Relaxation

Warm, moist air helps open stuffy bronchial and nasal passages. Lavender, rosemary, and bergamot aid in relaxing overworked throat and facial muscles while reducing the body's viral load.

```
3 cups steaming water
5 drops lavender essential oil
5 drops bergamot essential oil
5 drops rosemary essential oil
Clean towel
```

Pour the water into a shallow bowl. Add the essential oils. Position your face over the bowl, and cover your head with a towel to create a tent; breathe deeply until the water cools. Come up for air every minute or so, as needed.

Natural Disinfectant Room Spray

When you're feeling concerned about the spread of airborne viruses, help make indoor environments healthier with this natural disinfectant room spray. Echinacea essential oil has powerful antiviral properties that make it the ideal choice for use in helping prevent the spread of cold and flu germs.

```
20 drops echinacea essential oil
10 drops tea tree essential oil
8 ounces distilled water
```

Blend the essential oils. Pour the water into a dark-colored glass spray bottle, and add the essential oils. Shake the bottle vigorously before each use. Simply mist the air in the rooms where you'll be spending time.

CUTS, BURNS, AND BRUISES

Cypress Healing Spray

Using a spray made with essential oils can help bruises heal faster. Cypress essential oil helps strengthen capillary walls, while geranium, lavender, helichrysum, and frankincense provide soothing relief.

```
15 drops geranium essential oil
8 drops lavender essential oil
5 drops cypress essential oil
3 drops helichrysum essential oil
2 drops frankincense essential oil
1 teaspoon grain alcohol (omit if cuts
    or scrapes are present)
1/2 ounce distilled water
```

Blend the essential oils and grain alcohol in a 1-ounce glass spray bottle. Add the water, leaving a small amount of space below the bottle's neck. Shake well before applying to bruised skin.

Echinacea Wound Wash

If you've suffered a minor cut or burn, use this wound wash to cleanse it and start the healing process. Both yarrow and echinacea essential oils prevent infections while promoting faster healing.

```
6 drops echinacea essential oil
6 drops yarrow essential oil
3 ounces distilled water
```

Blend the essential oils, and then add them and the distilled water to a dark-colored spray bottle. Apply the mixture to affected areas as needed. Keep the bottle in the refrigerator for up to 6 months.

Healing Salve

If you've cut or burned yourself and need immediate relief, this healing salve will prove soothing. The yarrow, lavender, and Roman chamomile essential oils it contains are all excellent for helping to prevent pain and speed healing. Please note that this recipe is intended for use on minor injuries only.

```
30 drops lavender essential oil
15 drops yarrow essential oil
15 drops Roman chamomile essential oil
```

Combine all the essential oils. This blend may be used neat on minor wounds. For a healing massage, add 5 drops of the blended oil to each teaspoon of carrier oil you use. When used in massage oil, this blend boosts the immune system. Try it if you're fighting a cold or flu.

Aromatherapy Blend for Bruises

....

If you've bumped yourself and see a bruise developing, you can help soothe the pain and diminish the bruise's appearance with this blend. Both marigold and helichrysum essential oils are excellent anti-inflammatories.

```
8 drops marigold essential oil
8 drops helichrysum essential oil
2 ounces carrier oil
```

Blend the essential oils. Add to the carrier oil of your choice, such as jojoba or sweet almond oil. Apply directly to bruised area once or twice daily.

Marigold Healing Balm

....

If you have sore muscles, a minor scrape, an insect bite, or a rash, you'll find this marigold healing balm wonderfully effective. The lavender and marigold essential oils soothe and protect skin while preventing bacterial buildup.

```
1 ounce shea butter
1 ounce beeswax
3 ounces carrier oil
20 drops lavender essential oil
6 drops marigold essential oil
```

Melt the shea butter, beeswax, and carrier oil of your choice together in a glass bowl over a double boiler. Blend the essential oils in a separate container, then add them to bowl. Pour the mixture into a small jar with a tight-fitting lid, but allow it to cool completely before placing the lid on the jar.

DRY, ITCHY, OR SUNBURNED SKIN

Lavender-Lemon Balm Facial Toner

If your face is chapped, sunburned, or very dry, this toner provides rapid relief. The lavender and lemon balm it contains have anti-inflammatory properties that soothe skin.

```
8 drops lavender essential oil
6 drops Melissa (lemon balm) essential oil
1/4 cup whole milk
```

Blend the essential oils and then mix them into milk. Apply the blend to clean skin with a cotton ball 2–3 times daily. Store in the refrigerator between uses.

Dry Skin Sauna Treatment

If you suffer from dry facial skin, you'll love the way this simple beauty treatment soothes and moisturizes your face. The chamomile essential oil used in this treatment helps regenerate skin and restore moisture balance.

```
Bowl of steaming water
2 drops chamomile essential oil
Clean towel
```

Place the bowl on a table where you can sit comfortably in a chair. Pour the water into the bowl and add the chamomile essential oil. Place your face over the bowl, and tent the towel over your head. Enjoy the soothing fragrance and moisturizing steam until the water cools and the vapors stop. Emerge for a breath of fresh air occasionally, if needed.

Soothing Sunburn Salve

If you suffer a sunburn, apply this salve for cool comfort and instant relief. The yarrow, chamomile, and lavender oils it contains alleviate pain while promoting healing, while the avocado oil and aloe vera gel rehydrate the skin.

```
12 drops lavender essential oil
4 drops chamomile essential oil
4 drops yarrow essential oil
2 teaspoons avocado oil
2 tablespoons aloe vera gel
```

Blend the essential oils, then add them to the avocado oil. Combine this mixture with the aloe vera gel. Apply this formula generously to the affected areas. If you'd like to make a larger batch of this blend, store it in a glass container inside the refrigerator for no more than 2 weeks.

Yarrow-Frankincense Itch Preventive

If you suffer from eczema or psoriasis, you'll find this itch preventive to be effective. Yarrow, frankincense, and palmarosa essential oils soothe the skin and promote rapid healing.

```
8 drops yarrow essential oil
8 drops palmarosa essential oil
4 drops frankincense essential oil
2 teaspoons kukui nut oil
2 teaspoons jojoba oil
```

Blend all the essential oils, and then add the mixture to the kukui nut and jojoba oils. Apply this formula to the affected areas as needed.

Athlete's Foot Rub

Athlete's foot is caused by a fungal infection that causes itching and peeling, flaky skin. The antifungal properties of lavender and tea tree oil kill the fungus, while the oils' anti-inflammatory properties soothe the itch and ease burning and inflammation.

```
6 drops tea tree oil
3 drops lavender oil
1 ounce carrier oil
```

Combine the essential oils to a carrier oil of your choice, mixing well. Use a cotton swab to apply the mixture to the affected areas 3 times daily. Put on a clean pair of cotton socks after each use. Once the infection has subsided, use this foot rub at least a few times weekly to inhibit future fungal growth.

Toenail Fungus Blend

Toenail fungus is sometimes itchy; at other times, it is simply embarrassing. The antifungal property clove oil possesses makes it the ideal choice for eliminating toenail fungus.

```
2 drops clove oil
1 ounce carrier oil
```

Blend the clove oil into a carrier oil of your choice. Wash and dry the affected toenail thoroughly, ensuring that the towel you use to dry the toenail does not come in contact with other nails. Using a dropper, apply 3 drops of the solution to the affected toenail; then use a cotton swab to spread the oil across the affected area. Repeat twice daily. Wash and dry your hands thoroughly after each treatment.

Soothing Echinacea Body Powder

....

If you suffer from itchy, sweaty feet or if hot weather has you sweating more than you would like, use this soothing echinacea body powder to stay dry and comfortable. The echinacea essential oil it contains inhibits bacterial growth and will heal any cracked skin or areas where a rash is present.

```
6 drops echinacea essential oil
3 drops yarrow essential oil
1/2 cup arrowroot powder
1/4 cup baking soda
```

Blend the essential oils. Mix the arrowroot powder and baking soda in a large bowl, blender, or food processor. Add the essential oils and mix thoroughly. Store the mixture in a sugar shaker for easy application; use at least once daily for best results.

Softening Foot Scrub

....

Feet are often neglected, and they're almost always overworked. Soften your feet and help prevent calluses from forming with this delightfully simple scrub. The marigold oil helps soften skin while preventing the irritation scrubbing sometimes causes.

```
2 teaspoons fine to medium sea salt
2 teaspoons carrier oil
10 drops marigold essential oil
```

Combine the salt and carrier oil of your choice; then add the marigold essential oil and blend well. Soak your feet in warm water for 10 minutes; then towel dry. Sit comfortably with your feet on a towel. Use a pumice stone to loosen hardened skin, and then apply the foot scrub. Massage it in well, paying particular attention to dry, overworked areas such as the heels and balls of your feet. Rinse feet well once massage is complete. If you will not be using the mixture immediately, store it in a sealed container in a dark, cool place.

Tension Headache

....

A tension headache feels as if constant pressure is being applied, particularly at the temples or around the back of the head and neck. These headaches are usually caused by contraction of the neck and scalp muscles, so relief comes quickly once these muscles have been relaxed. Both peppermint and eucalyptus essential oils contain compounds that aid in muscle relaxation; combining these oils makes them even more effective.

```
10 drops peppermint essential oil
10 drops eucalyptus essential oil
20 drops carrier oil
```

Combine the essential oils with a carrier oil of your choice. Directly inhale, taking 3 slow, deep breaths. Next, massage a small amount of the blend into the skin at the back of your neck, using slow, deep strokes. Go all the way from the base of your skull to the point where your neck meets your shoulders. Massage a small amount into the temple area as well. Relax for several minutes, if possible. Repeat hourly as needed.

Cluster Headache

....

If you have recurring headaches characterized by throbbing pain on one side of your head, you may be suffering from cluster headaches. These are often accompanied by congestion on the same side as the pain, and relieving that congestion with peppermint essential oil while increasing blood circulation with frankincense essential oil can bring almost immediate relief.

```
2 drops frankincense essential oil
2 drops carrier oil
2 drops peppermint essential oil
Bowl of steaming water
Clean towel
```

Begin by blending the frankincense essential oil with a carrier oil of your choice. Massage two drops of this mixture into the sole of each foot.

Next, add the peppermint essential oil to the water. Tent the towel over your head and the bowl, and inhale the vapors deeply. Do this for 1–3 minutes. Relax afterward, and repeat again in 1 hour, if necessary.

Sinus Headache

When sinuses become inflamed, they can cause head pain, which is often accompanied by a fever. If you have a sinus infection, you may need antibiotics; in the meantime, you can soothe your headache by taking advantage of the powerful anti-inflammatory properties of eucalyptus and spearmint essential oils.

```
4 drops spearmint essential oil
4 drops eucalyptus essential oil
1 ounce carrier oil
```

Combine the essential oils with a carrier oil of your choice in a bottle. Warm the mixture by rolling the bottle between the palms of your hands. Massage your forehead and temples with 4 drops of the blend, and apply another 4 drops to the back of your neck near the base of your skull. This mixture is also excellent for diffusing and for direct inhalation.

Rebound Headache

....

Overuse of over-the-counter remedies for headaches and body aches can lead to rebound headaches. Common culprits include acetaminophen (Tylenol), aspirin, and ibuprofen. Select the appropriate headache remedies from this chapter to deal with the pain in your head, and detoxify your body to eliminate the chemicals that are causing your discomfort. Grapefruit, juniper, cypress, and laurel essential oils have powerful detoxification properties.

```
4 drops cypress essential oil
4 drops grapefruit essential oil
4 drops juniper essential oil
4 drops laurel essential oil
2 teaspoons carrier oil
```

Blend all the essential oils with a carrier oil of your choice. Gently massage the mixture onto your neck, armpits, feet, and the area behind your knees. Relax and drink plenty of water. To enhance the detoxification effect, add 1 drop of lemon essential oil to each glass of water that you drink.

Migraine

Migraines typically last between four and seventy-two hours, and are often accompanied by nausea, vomiting, or both, as well as sensitivity to light and noise. Directly inhaling peppermint or ginger essential oils can help ease nausea and take the edge off the headache; Roman chamomile and lavender essential oils have anti-inflammatory and sedative properties that ease pain while encouraging relaxation.

```
8 drops lavender essential oil
4 drops Roman chamomile essential oil
1 ounce carrier oil
```

Blend the essential oils with a carrier oil of your choice. Massage the temples, forehead, and back of the neck with the blend, and relax in a dark, cool, quiet place. To enhance this treatment, diffuse a few drops of the blend nearby.

LIVER CLEANSE

Body Detox

The liver has a tough job; it works hard to clear toxins from our bodies and can easily become inflamed. Lemon essential oil aids in clearing liver congestion and reducing toxic buildup, while peppermint essential oil encourages lymph drainage.

```
1 tablespoon freshly squeezed lemon juice
1 drop peppermint essential oil
1 drop lemon essential oil
```

Mix all the ingredients together in a glass of water; if you prefer, you can use more than 1 tablespoon of lemon juice. Drink the water all at once rather than sipping. Repeat once daily to help improve liver function.

Hangover Relief

....

*It's never a good idea to overdo it, but if you find yourself suffering a
hangover, cleansing your liver will help alleviate other symptoms rapidly.
Ginger essential oil helps soothe nausea, while lemon essential oil aids in
clearing toxins fast. Pair this remedy with a headache-relief treatment for
whole-body hangover relief.*

```
1 tablespoon freshly squeezed lemon juice
1 drop ginger essential oil
1 drop lemon essential oil
```

Blend all the ingredients together in a glass of water. Drink it down all at
once. Repeat in 1 hour if needed.

MUSCLE PAIN

Injury or Trauma

....

*Remembering that essential oils are not a substitute for medical care but
a complement to it, you can put this remedy to work to help alleviate pain
from a muscle injury or trauma. Cold compresses help reduce swelling,
and when combined with marjoram, basil, and citronella essential oils, all
of which have anti-inflammatory properties, they bring soothing relief.*

```
1 pint ice-cold water
4 drops sweet marjoram essential oil
4 drops citronella essential oil
1 drop basil essential oil
Clean towel
```

Blend all the ingredients together in a bowl or basin. Soak a soft flannel cloth
or terry towel in the mixture and apply to injured area. Repeat as cloth warms
from body heat.

Muscle Overuse

If you've overused muscles, pain and stiffness caused by a buildup of lactic acid (which causes muscle fibers to stick together) can result. Gently massaging sore muscles helps; adding anti-inflammatory essential oils speeds relief.

```
7 drops lavender essential oil
5 drops Scots pine essential oil
3 drops eucalyptus essential oil
2 ounces carrier oil
```

Blend all the essential oils with a carrier oil of your choice in a bottle. Warm the mixture by rolling the bottle between the palms of your hands. Gently massage the affected area, using just enough oil to penetrate the skin. Repeat as needed.

Stress, Anxiety, and Tension

When life's stresses take over, muscles often become tight and painful. Using a muscle-relaxing combination of heat and aromatherapy provides relief while easing stress.

```
4 drops rosemary essential oil
3 drops sweet marjoram essential oil
2 drops Roman chamomile essential oil
```

Fill your bathtub with hot water and add the essential oils. If you like, you can diffuse lavender essential oil in the bathroom to intensify relaxation. If possible, take a nap after bathing.

Relaxing Muscle Soak

If you've got sore muscles, whether from a day of hiking through the woods or from a day of sitting in an office chair, you'll appreciate this soothing chamomile soak. The lavender, chamomile, and clary sage essential oils promote relaxation while quieting the mind in preparation for a good night's sleep.

```
10 drops chamomile essential oil
7 drops lavender essential oil
5 drops Roman chamomile essential oil
2 drops clary sage essential oil
15 drops carrier oil
```

Blend all the essential oils with a carrier oil of your choice. Draw a hot bath. Add the essential oil blend to the bath, step in, and relax.

General Aches and Pains

Use this simple recipe to soothe general aches and pains. The peppermint essential oil combines with the lavender, cedar, and oregano essential oils to provide cool, soothing relief.

```
2 drops lavender essential oil
2 drops cedarwood essential oil
3 drops oregano essential oil
4 drops peppermint essential oil
1 tablespoon carrier oil
```

Blend essential oils; combine with carrier oil. Apply to affected area as needed, using small circular motions to massage into skin.

Indigestion

If you are suffering from indigestion and are feeling nauseous, you'll find the following remedy effective. The menthol in peppermint oil improves circulation and stops nausea rapidly.

```
3 drops peppermint essential oil
Clean cloth or facial tissue
```

Drip 3 drops of peppermint essential oil onto the cloth or facial tissue. Hold it under your nose, being careful not to allow the oil to contact your skin. Breathe slowly and deeply for 1–3 minutes.

Motion Sickness

When suffering nausea and vomiting as the result of motion sickness, spearmint essential oil provides rapid comfort, thanks to its antispasmodic property.

```
2 drops spearmint essential oil
4 drops carrier oil
```

Combine the essential oil and carrier oil of your choice, and massage the mixture onto the mastoid area behind each ear once hourly while traveling. You may also directly inhale the spearmint oil or place 1–4 drops of the diluted oil directly onto your tongue.

Vomiting

....

If you are vomiting or feel that you may begin vomiting, patchouli is one of the best oils to use, as the compounds the oil contains reduce the strength of gastrointestinal muscle contractions.

```
Patchouli essential oil, undiluted
```

If able, place 1–4 drops of patchouli essential oil directly onto your tongue. You may also directly inhale the oil 4–6 times per hour or as needed.

Stomach Flu

....

With the stomach flu comes nausea, fever, headaches, and vomiting. Ginger essential oil reduces fever and nausea, while lavender oil is a strong antiseptic. Both peppermint and spearmint help ease nausea.

```
4 drops ginger essential oil
2 drops lavender essential oil
1 drop peppermint essential oil
1 drop spearmint essential oil
8 drops carrier oil
```

Combine the essential oils with a carrier oil of your choice. This blend may be directly inhaled, diffused, or applied to the mastoids behind each ear once every hour. If you have only peppermint or spearmint essential oil, simply use 2 drops of the oil you have on hand to complete this recipe.

Morning Sickness

When suffering from morning sickness, safe, natural remedies are best. Lemon and ginger essential oils are safe for use during pregnancy and are effective in combating nausea.

```
4 drops lemon essential oil
4 drops ginger essential oil
8 drops carrier oil
```

Blend the essential oils with a carrier oil of your choice; diffuse in the area where you spend the most time. You can also blend the oils and inhale them directly from a handkerchief or vial.

CHAPTER SIX

Essential Oils for Enhanced Well-Being

CALM

Balancing Lavender Aromatherapy Blend

....

When tension needs taming, this balancing lavender aromatherapy blend calms and refreshes. Juniper, bergamot, and patchouli essential oils promote peaceful feelings, while lavender has a slight sedative effect that helps take the edge off.

```
14 drops bergamot essential oil
14 drops lavender essential oil
2 drops juniper essential oil
2 drops patchouli essential oil
```

Combine all the essential oils, and diffuse or blend them with water for a room spray. This blend is also a fantastic addition to a bath; add 4 drops to the tub and relax.

Refreshing Vanilla-Rose Body Spray

....

Enjoy a sense of calm that lasts all day with this delightful antibacterial body spray. Not only do rose otto and lavender essential oils prevent body odor, they promote a sense of calm, while the vanilla helps enhance mood and bring on a feeling of total well-being.

```
12 drops rose otto essential oil
3 drops lavender essential oil
1 drop vanilla essential oil
1 ounce distilled water
```

Combine all the oils, then mix them with the water in a small spray bottle. Spritz the blend onto bare skin after showering or bathing.

Calming Sandalwood Soak

....

When worries and anxiety take over, sandalwood and ylang-ylang can aid in centering the mind and releasing anxious thoughts. Enjoy this soak anytime nervousness or tension arises.

```
4 drops sandalwood essential oil
1 drop ylang-ylang essential oil
```

Add the essential oils to a warm bath. Enjoy the calming vapors while relaxing and allowing your mind to drift.

Calming Commuter's Spray

If driving in traffic leaves you feeling tense and edgy, try this calming spray in the car. It's fantastic for home and office use, too. The lavender calms tension, while geranium and clary sage promote balance. Peppermint lifts the spirits.

```
3 drops lavender essential oil
1 drop clary sage essential oil
1 drop geranium essential oil
1 drop peppermint essential oil
1 ounce distilled water
```

Combine all the essential oils. Blend them with the distilled water in a spray bottle. Shake well and spritz car interior prior to commute or during traffic jams.

Calming Vanilla Mist

Whether you need to relax at bedtime or you simply want to indulge in a relaxing, all-natural air freshener with no added chemicals, you'll enjoy this calming vanilla mist. The lavender and chamomile it contains soothes a busy mind and promotes relaxation.

```
15 drops chamomile essential oil
15 drops lavender essential oil
4 drops vanilla essential oil
6 ounces distilled water
```

Blend the essential oils; add them to the water in a glass spray bottle. Shake well before spritzing the mixture into the air.

Mentally Soothing Aromatherapy Blend

When your mind is overworked or troubled, try this mentally soothing aromatherapy blend. Lavender, sandalwood, and neroli essential oils promote feelings of calm, while rose otto, jasmine, and vanilla promote overall feelings of well-being.

```
10 drops jasmine essential oil
10 drops rose otto essential oil
4 drops lavender essential oil
2 drops neroli essential oil
2 drops sandalwood essential oil
2 drops vanilla essential oil
```

Blend all the essential oils. Add them to 2 ounces of your favorite massage oil, diffuse, or add to an 8-ounce spray bottle filled with distilled water for enjoyment anytime.

DEPRESSION

Vanilla-Jasmine Mist

If you're feeling low, this beautifully scented mist can lift your spirits. Both vanilla and jasmine are renowned for their ability to help relieve depression.

```
4 drops jasmine essential oil
1 drop vanilla essential oil
4 ounces distilled water
```

Blend the essential oils; add them to the water in a spray bottle. Use the mist to spritz yourself after showering and to freshen indoor spaces.

Chamomile-Bergamot Aromatherapy Blend

Depression can bring feelings of bitterness and anger with it. If you are brooding and feeling moody, this aromatherapy blend can help. Chamomile, bergamot, and helichrysum alleviate feelings of anger while helping the mind relax.

```
3 drops bergamot essential oil
3 drops helichrysum essential oil
3 drops Roman chamomile essential oil
```

Blend the essential oils and diffuse. For a portable spray you can enjoy anytime, add to a 1-ounce spray bottle filled with distilled water.

Soothing Sandalwood-Vanilla Soak

When feelings of depression threaten, relaxing the body and mind can work wonders. Vanilla is renowned for its uplifting fragrance, while sandalwood and chamomile relax the body and mind.

```
4 drops Roman chamomile essential oil
4 drops sandalwood essential oil
1 drop vanilla essential oil
```

Blend all the essential oils; then add them to a hot bath. Relax and breathe deeply. This blend may also be diffused or added to a 1-ounce spray bottle filled with distilled water for a portable remedy.

Citrus-Sage Aromatherapy Rub

A soothing temple massage helps relax the mind and stop negative thought patterns. Orange essential oil brightens gloomy moods, while clary sage is renowned for its ability to ease depression and put a stop to melancholy thoughts.

```
9 drops orange essential oil
6 drops clary sage essential oil
```

Blend the essential oils. Apply 1–2 drops to each temple then massage slowly. This blend is also useful for diffusion and may be added to a 1-ounce spray bottle filled with distilled water for an uplifting aromatherapy mist.

Ylang-Ylang Citrus Aromatherapy Rub

When feeling depressed, motivation can be hard to come by. Ylang-ylang, grapefruit, and bergamot essential oils lift the spirits while providing a welcome energy boost.

```
9 drops bergamot essential oil
3 drops grapefruit essential oil
3 drops ylang-ylang essential oil
```

Blend all the essential oils. Apply 3–4 drops to your fingertips; then massage the back of your neck from the base of your skull to your shoulders. This rub may also be applied to the temples or the mastoids. It is also suitable for diffusion, and may be added to a 1-ounce spray bottle filled with distilled water for an uplifting room mist.

Ylang-Ylang Mist

....

*When things aren't going well, give your mood an instant boost with this mist.
Ylang-ylang promotes relaxation and helps relieve tension, while orange
helps promote happiness.*

```
12 drops orange essential oil
5 drops ylang-ylang essential oil
3 drops peppermint essential oil
4 ounces distilled water
```

Combine the essential oils and water in a spray bottle. Shake vigorously and
spritz for sweet-smelling air and an instant attitude adjustment.

Spruce Diffusion

....

*If you're feeling irritable, elevate your mood with this spruce diffusion. If
you don't have spruce essential oil, Scots pine or fir needle can be used in its
place. The alpha-pinene these evergreens contain helps relax the mind.*

```
5 drops spruce essential oil
1 drop basil essential oil
1 drop bergamot essential oil
7 drops carrier oil
```

Blend the essential oils with a carrier oil of your choice and diffuse. If you
prefer, skip the carrier oil and blend the essential oils with four ounces of
distilled water for an equally uplifting room spray.

Focus-Enhancing Temple Massage

When you're feeling out of sorts and can't seem to focus, enhance concentration with this soothing temple massage. Bergamot helps improve circulation, and both bergamot and clary sage aid in elevating mood.

```
3 drops bergamot essential oil
3 drops clary sage essential oil
1 tablespoon carrier oil
```

Combine the essential oils with a carrier oil of your choice; then massage your temples with 2 drops of the blend. Close your eyes and inhale. You'll feel better in a few moments.

Geranium-Lavender Balancing Blend

If you are suffering from an unpleasant mood, this balancing aromatherapy blend can help set things right. Geranium normalizes mood and promotes balance, while lavender, bergamot, and rose otto promote feelings of well-being.

```
20 drops geranium essential oil
15 drops lavender essential oil
10 drops bergamot essential oil
5 drops rose otto essential oil
```

Combine all the essential oils and diffuse. For faster results, blend the essential oils and a small amount of water in a spray bottle and spritz throughout your home or office.

Emotional Release Aromatherapy Blend

....

When pent-up emotions are causing a gloomy mood, this emotionally cleansing aromatherapy blend can alleviate tension. Grapefruit's fragrance melts moodiness, while rose otto and bergamot promote emotional balance.

```
4-5 drops grapefruit essential oil
3 drops bergamot essential oil
3 drops rose otto essential oil
```

Combine the essential oils. Diffuse 6 drops at a time, or blend with distilled water in an 8-ounce spray bottle to use anytime emotional tension arises.

STRESS

Stress-Free Soak

....

After a stressful day at work, there's nothing quite like a warm aromatherapy bath to relieve tension. The lavender in this blend aids in relaxation, while the bergamot and coriander relieve stress and boost the spirits.

```
15 drops lavender essential oil
2 drops bergamot essential oil
2 drops coriander essential oil
1 drop patchouli essential oil
1 teaspoon carrier oil
1/2 cup Dead Sea salt
```

Blend the essential oils; add them to a carrier oil of your choice. Mix in the salt and place the blend in a container with a tight-fitting lid. Use 2 tablespoons at a time.

Aromatherapy Foot Massage Blend

When stress takes its toll, the feet are often last to receive care. This refreshing foot massage blend uses tea tree and peppermint essential oils to invigorate the mind and soothe tired feet.

```
6 drops peppermint essential oil
6 drops tea tree essential oil
1 ounce carrier oil
```

Blend the essential oils; add them to a carrier oil of your choice. Massage the blend into your feet, paying particular attention to your toes and arches.

Soothing Vanilla Body Moisturizer

Some scents can help keep stress at bay all day. In this delicious-smelling blend, orange and vanilla essential oils come together to ease tension and promote positive thoughts.

```
10 drops orange essential oil
2 drops vanilla essential oil
2 ounces carrier oil
```

Blend the essential oils; add them to a carrier oil of your choice. Store the mixture in a dark-colored glass bottle, and smooth onto body after bathing or showering.

Stress-Free Aromatherapy Blend

Maintaining a positive frame of mind can help keep stress at bay. This aromatherapy blend relies on a trio of uplifting essential oils.

```
6 drops bergamot essential oil
6 drops clary sage essential oil
3 drops frankincense essential oil
```

Mix the essential oils together. This blend may be applied to the temples, diffused, or added to a 1-ounce spray bottle filled with distilled water.

Citrus-Frankincense Aromatherapy Blend

If you are feeling stressed and agitated or angry, this aromatherapy blend can help restore good spirits. Lemon, frankincense, and neroli are all natural mood boosters.

```
6 drops frankincense essential oil
3 drops lemon essential oil
3 drops neroli essential oil
```

Mix the essential oils together. This blend may be applied to the temples, diffused, or added to a 1-ounce spray bottle filled with distilled water.

Uplifting Body and Bath Oil

Lift your spirits and release tension with this uplifting body and bath oil. The geranium essential oil in this recipe promotes balance, while the lavender eases tension and the lemongrass lifts the spirits.

```
10 drops geranium essential oil
9 drops lavender essential oil
7 drops lemongrass essential oil
4 ounces carrier oil
```

Blend the essential oils with a carrier oil of your choice. Use 2 tablespoons in a warm bath, or apply a small amount to damp skin after a hot shower.

Refreshing Basil Aromatherapy Blend

When physical and emotional fatigue take their toll, this rejuvenating basil aromatherapy blend helps restore balance. Basil essential oil inspires positive thinking and promotes clarity.

```
20 drops basil essential oil
20 drops bergamot essential oil
7 drops peppermint essential oil
5 drops lavender essential oil
3 drops eucalyptus essential oil
```

Combine the essential oils and diffuse 12 drops at a time. Alternatively, add the mixture to distilled water in an 8-ounce spray bottle for a refreshing room spray.

Energizing Liquid Body Cleanser

··

Uplift your spirits while showering with this delightfully energizing liquid body cleanser. When combined with peppermint, lavender lifts the spirits. Cypress adds balance to this invigorating blend.

```
28 drops cypress essential oil
16 drops lavender essential oil
4 drops peppermint essential oil
8 ounces unscented liquid body soap
```

Combine all the essential oils; add them to the body soap. Stir vigorously until well blended. Pour a small amount on a shower pouf and enjoy.

Eucalyptus Energy Spritz

··

Uplift your spirits and invigorate your mind with this irresistible eucalyptus energy spritz. The combination of lemon, lavender, eucalyptus, spearmint, and petitgrain can jump-start creativity while providing a cool, tingling sensation.

```
20 drops lavender essential oil
10 drops eucalyptus essential oil
10 drops lemon essential oil
5 drops petitgrain essential oil
5 drops spearmint essential oil
6 ounces distilled water
```

Combine all the essential oils, then add them to the distilled water in a spray bottle with an atomizer. (A spray bottle will work as an acceptable substitute for an atomizer, if you like.) Use this blend as a body mist after showering or anytime you need a pick-me-up.

Uplifting Aromatherapy Diffusion

Enjoy a mental boost with this energizing blend. Lavender, mandarin, and bergamot combine to lift the spirits with a fresh, summery aroma.

```
16 drops bergamot essential oil
16 drops lavender essential oil
8 drops mandarin essential oil
```

Combine the essential oils. Diffuse to bring an instant aura of cheer to any setting, or add to 8 ounces of distilled water for an energizing room spray.

CHAPTER SEVEN

Cosmetic Uses of Essential Oils

DEODORANT

Lavender Deodorant Spray

Perspiration takes on an unpleasant odor due to bacterial growth. The lavender essential oil in this deodorant spray inhibits bacteria and keeps you smelling fresh.

```
20 drops lavender essential oil
4 ounces distilled water
```

Blend the essential oil with the distilled water in a spray bottle. Apply the mixture to your entire body after showering.

Nontoxic Underarm Deodorant

If you want to eliminate toxins from your daily routine, rethinking your deodorant makes a difference. The essential oils in this deodorant recipe inhibit bacterial growth and smell fantastic. You will need a 10-milliliter bottle with a roll-on cap. If one is not available, you can swab the deodorant on with a cotton ball; however, you'll end up using a lot more that way.

50 drops clary sage essential oil
50 drops lavender essential oil
15 drops patchouli essential oil
12 drops frankincense essential oil

Blend all the essential oils together in the roll-on bottle, and apply to underarm area as needed.

Absorbent Underarm Deodorant

If you don't like the idea of applying toxic aluminum to your underarms daily, give this absorbent underarm deodorant a try. The baking soda and cornstarch it contains absorb wetness and odor, while the essential oils have antifungal and antibacterial properties to keep you smelling fresh.

```
4 tablespoons organic unrefined extra-virgin coconut oil
5 drops lavender essential oil
5 drops tea tree essential oil
4 tablespoons cornstarch
4 tablespoons baking soda
```

Melt the coconut oil in a glass bowl, and allow it to cool until just warm. Blend the essential oils together and combine them with the coconut oil, mixing well. Mix the cornstarch and baking soda together in a second glass bowl. Add the oil blend to the dry ingredients and mix thoroughly. Place the resulting paste into a glass jar with a tight-fitting lid, but allow it to cool naturally with the lid off before capping the jar. Store the deodorant in the refrigerator. Apply it to clean underarms with your fingertips, taking care to use only a small amount.

Deodorizing Body Powder

If you suffer from sweaty feet or excessive perspiration, you'll enjoy this simple, effective deodorizing body powder. The cornstarch and baking soda absorb moisture and stop odor, while the essential oils inhibit bacterial growth.

```
1/2 cup cornstarch or arrowroot powder
1/3 cup baking soda
3 drops lavender essential oil
2 drops rosemary essential oil
```

Mix the dry ingredients together in a glass bowl. Blend the essential oils together, then add them to the dry ingredients. Store the mixture in a glass jar or sugar shaker. To apply to underarms, pat on with a slightly damp washcloth. For use on feet, simply sprinkle a small amount into your socks or shoes.

HAIR

Stimulating Rosemary-Mint Shampoo

Wake up with the invigorating fragrance of rosemary mint shampoo. Peppermint provides a cooling sensation, while rosemary increases circulation. Both are excellent tonics for the scalp.

```
6 drops rosemary essential oil
3 drops peppermint essential oil
8 ounces unscented shampoo
```

Combine the essential oils and add them to the shampoo. Blend thoroughly, work up a lather, and rinse.

Lavender-Tea Tree Dandruff Shampoo

Do you suffer from dandruff? This refreshing shampoo combines two potent essential oils known for their ability to address skin problems. Its fragrance is fresh and invigorating, so you'll enjoy using it every time you shower.

```
10 drops lavender essential oil
4 drops tea tree essential oil
8 ounces unscented shampoo
```

Combine the essential oils and add them to the shampoo. Blend thoroughly, work up a lather, and allow to rest on the scalp for at least 30 seconds. Rinse.

Nourishing Helichrysum-Cypress Shampoo

Add shine and an irresistible scent to your hair with this delightful shampoo. Helichrysum is known for its healing properties, and cypress helps remove excess oil without stripping hair.

```
6 drops cypress essential oil
6 drops helichrysum essential oil
8 ounces unscented shampoo
```

Combine the essential oils; then add them to the shampoo. Blend thoroughly, work up a lather, and enjoy.

Softening Lavender-Rosemary Conditioner

This conditioner is ideal for all hair types. Lavender soothes the scalp, while rosemary prevents excess oil buildup.

```
6 drops lavender essential oil
6 drops rosemary essential oil
8 ounces unscented conditioner
```

Combine the essential oils and blend them with the conditioner. Apply the mixture to your hair after shampooing and rinsing. Allow it to sit for 30–60 seconds, rinse thoroughly.

Oily Hair Remedy

If you have oily hair, try this blend before shampooing. Cedar essential oil is an excellent astringent that helps remove excess oils without stripping the hair.

```
6 drops cedarwood essential oil
2 drops rosemary essential oil
2 teaspoons olive oil
```

Combine all the oils. Massage the mixture into your scalp, and allow to sit for 1–3 minutes before shampooing.

Invigorating Massage Blend

....

Soften skin and soothe tired muscles with this invigorating blend. Pepper-mint, wintergreen, and clove help improve circulation, which nourishes your skin from the inside out.

```
30 drops German chamomile essential oil
10 drops Roman chamomile essential oil
6 drops peppermint essential oil
4 drops wintergreen essential oil
2 drops clove essential oil
2 ounces carrier oil
```

Blend all the essential oils and add the mixture to a carrier oil of your choice. Massage the blend into your skin. Avoid contact with your eyes and other sensitive areas. As with all products containing wintergreen, do not use on children or pregnant women, or those with aspirin sensitivities. (See page 146 for a list of interactions).

Healing Wintertime Body Moisturizer

If you have dry, irritated skin, this body moisturizer will leave it feeling soft and supple. Myrrh is renowned for its healing qualities and has a wonderful fragrance most people enjoy, while orange nourishes skin and provides an uplifting quality to the moisturizer's aroma.

```
10 drops myrrh essential oil
10 drops orange essential oil
16 ounces sweet almond oil
4 ounces cocoa butter
```

Blend the essential oils, then combine them with the sweet almond oil. Melt the cocoa butter in a saucepan, using low heat. Once melted, add the oil blend and mix thoroughly. Pour the mixture into a container, and allow to cool before capping with a tight-fitting lid. If using immediately, allow to cool before use.

Orange-Jasmine Body Spa

If you have some time to spare and want to pamper your skin, try this body spa treatment. Jasmine, sandalwood, and orange oils soften the skin, while the fragrance calms and uplifts the mind.

```
10 drops orange essential oil
6 drops sandalwood essential oil
4 drops jasmine essential oil
1 tablespoon jojoba oil
```

Combine all the essential oils, and blend them with the jojoba oil. Add the mixture to a steaming bath, slip in, and relax.

Rose Spa Facial

....

If you're feeling tired and need a boost, try this spa facial. Though simple, it works wonders for tired skin, thanks to the rose otto essential oil's ability to moisturize and renew even the driest skin.

```
5 drops rose otto essential oil
```

Apply the rose otto essential oil directly to the palm of your hand. Use your fingers to gently apply it to your face and neck. Use a warm, moist washcloth to cover your face and keep it there until it cools.

Purifying Bergamot Face Mask

....

If you have oily skin, you'll enjoy using this face mask to remove excess oil and increase smoothness. Lavender, bergamot, and clary sage help remove excess oil without stripping skin.

```
8 drops lavender essential oil
4 drops bergamot essential oil
3 drops clary sage essential oil
2 tablespoons cornmeal
2 tablespoons raw almond meal
2–3 tablespoons water
```

Blend the essential oils together. Mix the cornmeal and almond meal together, then add the essential oils. Add water gradually until a paste forms. Apply the mixture to your face, using a gentle circular motion. Allow it to dry, then rinse your face with warm water. Pat your face dry with a soft towel.

Rejuvenating Neroli Face Mask

If your face looks tired, this rejuvenating face mask will provide you with a boost. Yogurt and neroli essential oil contain amino acids that help build and maintain skin's collagen cells.

5 drops neroli essential oil

2 tablespoons unflavored organic yogurt

Blend the essential oil into the yogurt, then apply the mixture to your face. Leave in place for 10 minutes; then rinse your face with lukewarm water and pat dry with a soft towel.

Moisturizing Citrus Face Mask

When your face feels dry, it's easy to moisturize it in just a few minutes with the help of this mask. Lemon and orange essential oils are hydrating and contain plenty of vitamin C, which your skin needs for good health.

$^1/_4$ avocado

3 drops orange essential oil

2 drops lemon essential oil

Mash the avocado thoroughly, then add the essential oils. Apply the mixture to your clean face, and allow it to sit for at least 10 minutes before rinsing it off with warm water and patting dry with a soft towel.

Exfoliating Rosemary Face Mask

If your skin often has a dull appearance, exfoliating on a regular basis can brighten it. Rosemary essential oil is an excellent moisturizer, and when paired with fresh citrus, it works wonders on dull, dry skin.

```
2 tablespoons cornmeal
2 tablespoons raw almond meal
Juice of 1 organic orange
5 drops rosemary essential oil
```

Mix the cornmeal and almond meal together. Add orange juice in small amounts until a spreadable paste forms. Add the essential oil and blend. Apply it to your face. Leave in place for 10 minutes, then rinse with lukewarm water and pat dry with a soft towel.

Moisturizing Rosemary Facial Toner

If you have dry skin, you'll appreciate this nondrying rosemary facial toner. Rosemary essential oil is an excellent natural moisturizer.

```
2 ounces witch hazel
10 drops rosemary essential oil
```

Blend witch hazel and the essential oil in a dark-colored glass bottle. Apply a small amount to your face with a cotton ball each morning and evening after cleansing. Follow up with moisturizer.

Invigorating Rosemary-Mint Facial Toner

If you are beginning to notice that your skin is aging, yet you battle the occasional breakout, you'll benefit from this invigorating facial toner. The wine contains alpha hydroxy acid, while the peppermint and rosemary essential oils work to moisturize and refresh.

½ cup white wine
10 drops rosemary essential oil
3 drops peppermint essential oil

Simmer the wine in a saucepan for 10 minutes. Allow it to cool until luke-warm. Add the essential oils, place the mixture in a 4-ounce bottle. Apply a small amount to clean skin with a cotton ball. Keep this blend refrigerated and use within 6 months.

Renewing Aloe-Lime Facial Toner

If your skin looks tired, dry, or dull, this renewing facial toner can make an improvement. Aloe vera hydrates and heals, while lime cleanses and gently exfoliates.

1 tablespoon aloe vera juice
3 drops lime essential oil

Blend the aloe vera juice and lime essential oil. Apply the mixture to your face with a clean cotton ball. Leave it in place for at least 10 minutes, then rinse with cool water.

Yarrow Toner for Oily Skin

If you have oily skin, try this toner. Your skin will feel cool, clear, and comfortable immediately after use, thanks to the yarrow essential oil and witch hazel. Don't be frightened by the boric acid. It is a very weak acid in a naturally occurring mineral form, which is often used in antiseptics. It is found in volcanic areas, and it is a constituent in many plants and almost all fruits.

```
2 tablespoons witch hazel
Pinch boric acid
3 ounces distilled water
3 drops yarrow essential oil
```

Blend the witch hazel with the boric acid, then add the distilled water and yarrow essential oil. Store the mixture in a glass bottle, and apply it to your face with a cotton ball as needed. If you prefer a cooling mist, you add a spray top to the storage bottle.

Soothing Facial Scrub

If you've got dry skin and need to exfoliate, but don't want to use harsh abrasives, you'll enjoy using this soothing facial scrub. The lavender and chamomile essential oils it contains soothe the skin while preventing irritation.

```
10 drops chamomile essential oil
10 drops lavender essential oil
1 ounce sweet almond oil or jojoba oil
1 tablespoon ground oat flour
2 tablespoons superfine sugar
```

Blend the essential oils and add them to the almond or jojoba oil. Combine the oat flour and sugar, then add the oils. Pat your face with warm water, then apply the scrub using firm circular motions. Rinse well and pat dry afterward.

Tamanu Shave Balm

Ideal for men and women alike, this shave balm provides soothing moisture after a shave. Choose high-quality, cold-pressed tamanu oil for best results.

```
12 drops chamomile essential oil
12 drops lavender essential oil
12 drops patchouli essential oil
1 tablespoon cold-pressed tamanu oil
1/2 cup aloe vera gel
```

Combine all the essential oils, then add them to the tamanu oil. Blend the oils with the aloe vera gel in a glass bowl. Place the mixture in a glass jar; store away from direct heat and out of sunlight. Apply the balm to damp skin after shaving.

SOAP

Nourishing Chamomile Body Wash

Roman chamomile and vanilla work wonders for dry, irritated skin while calming the spirit and leaving a fresh, pleasant scent behind.

```
6 drops Roman chamomile essential oil
6 drops vanilla essential oil
8 ounces unscented body wash
```

Combine the essential oils; blend with the body wash. Apply a small amount to a bath pouf and enjoy.

Sensual Neroli-Sandalwood Sugar Scrub

Treat yourself to an exfoliating sugar scrub that leaves the skin feeling smooth and soft. Neroli, sandalwood, vanilla, and orange essential oils lift the spirits.

```
3 drops neroli essential oil
3 drops orange essential oil
3 drops sandalwood essential oil
3 drops vanilla essential oil
1 ounce carrier oil
1/2 cup organic cane sugar
```

Blend the essential oils; add them to a carrier oil of your choice. Add the sugar and mix thoroughly. Use immediately or store in an airtight container for up to 6 months.

Refreshing Herbal Shower Gel

Shake off sleep and prepare for the day ahead with this invigorating shower gel. Peppermint and eucalyptus feel refreshing to the skin, while ginger and orange nourish.

```
40 drops peppermint essential oil
12 drops eucalyptus essential oil
12 drops orange essential oil
8 drops ginger essential oil
8 ounces unscented shower gel
```

Combine the essential oils, then add them to the shower gel. Mix thoroughly. Apply a small amount to a shower pouf and enjoy.

Relaxing Body Wash

....

A warm shower can help you relax at bedtime. Lavender and chamomile have potent sedative properties, so sleep comes easier.

```
10 drops chamomile essential oil
10 drops lavender essential oil
8 ounces unscented liquid body wash
```

Combine the essential oils; add them to the body wash and blend well. Apply a small amount to a shower pouf and enjoy.

CHAPTER EIGHT

Essential Oils for Home and Garden

AIR FRESHENERS

Homemade Reed Diffuser

··

Commercially produced reed diffusers rely on chemicals to provide fragrance. If you'd like a nontoxic alternative, take a few minutes to make this fantastic homemade reed diffuser. The small jars used here can be found at a craft store.

```
Small jar with cork lid
Bamboo barbecue skewers
15 drops essential oil or essential oil blend
Carrier oil
1 teaspoon rubbing alcohol or vodka
```

Drill or punch a hole in the center of the jar's cork to make room for a few bamboo barbecue skewers.

Fill the jar about ⅓ full with carrier oil. Safflower oil is a good alternative to more expensive carriers; the lighter the oil, the easier it will be for the fragrance to travel up the reeds.

Blend your favorite essential oils into the carrier oil. Choose one of the blends in this book to achieve specific therapeutic results. Add rubbing alcohol or vodka to the blend; this helps the fragrance travel up the reeds.

Cork the bottle and add 3–4 barbecue skewers. Tie raffia or a ribbon around the bottle's neck for a decorative touch.

Gel Air Freshener

If you love clean-smelling indoor spaces but hate chemicals, you'll enjoy using this simple gel air freshener in place of toxic commercially produced types.

```
1 cup water
1 ounce plain powdered gelatin
1 tablespoon table salt
2 small glass jars
30 drops essential oil or essential oil blend
```

Bring the water to a boil in a small saucepan, and add the powdered gelatin. Whisk until smooth. Add the salt and whisk until it is dissolved, then remove it from the heat.

Prepare the glass jars by sprinkling your favorite essential oil into the bottom of each—use a blend from this book, if you like. Pour the hot gelatin into the jars. Allow the mixture to cool before placing wherever a fresh scent is needed.

Quick Air-Freshening Granules

Commercially produced air-freshening granules are convenient, but they contain toxic ingredients. Use this simple recipe to create nontoxic air-freshening granules that emit a fresh, lasting fragrance.

Small glass jar
Uncooked rice
10–20 drops essential oil or essential oil blend

Fill a small jar with any type of uncooked rice. Add your favorite essential oil and blend well. Place the scented rice wherever a fresh scent is appreciated. Try lavender in the bedroom, mint and lemon in the bathroom, or clary sage and orange in the kitchen.

Easy Odor-Stopping Air Freshener

Stop odor without resorting to the use of commercially produced air fresheners that contain toxic ingredients. The baking soda in this recipe absorbs odors, while the citrus essential oils freshen the air.

Sugar shaker
Baking soda
30 drops orange essential oil
20 drops lemon essential oil

Fill a sugar shaker or large salt shaker ⅓ full with baking soda. Add the essential oils and blend thoroughly. Replace the cap and set the shaker in an area that requires freshening. This recipe is very nice for use in the refrigerator, behind garbage cans, and in closets where smelly gym equipment is stored.

Air Freshening Spray

To give your home a fast fragrance boost, skip toxic sprays in favor of this simple homemade air freshening spray. Choose your favorite aromatherapy blend to reap the benefits of essential oils.

³/₄ cup distilled water
8-ounce spray bottle
1¹/₂ tablespoons vodka
20 drops essential oil or essential oil blend

Pour the distilled water into the spray bottle. Add the vodka and the essential oil. Shake vigorously before each use.

Refreshing Green Tea Bug Lotion

This lotion protects and moisturizes, and is excellent for all skin types. Geranium, grapefruit, and lavender essential oils nourish skin, while eucalyptus helps keep bugs at bay.

3/4 ounce beeswax

1 cup sweet almond oil

28 drops eucalyptus essential oil

6 drops lavender essential oil

4 drops grapefruit essential oil

2 drops geranium essential oil

1 cup lukewarm green tea

Place the beeswax and almond oil in a glass container, and melt the mixture over a double boiler. Allow it to cool until lukewarm. Pour the green tea into a blender, mixer, or food processor. Turn the machine on, and add the oil mixture in a thin stream. Blend until the mixture takes on a creamy appearance. Add the essential oils and blend. Store in a jar with a tight-fitting lid. Refrigerate to preserve the essential oils for a longer period of time. Mixture will stay fresh for up to 2 weeks.

Natural Mosquito Repellent

....

If you enjoy the outdoors but hate being bitten by bugs, this mosquito repellent is a great alternative to dangerous chemical insect repellents. All the essential oils it contains are natural insect deterrents.

```
20 drops lemongrass essential oil
20 drops citronella essential oil
5 drops tea tree essential oil
10 drops rosemary essential oil
1½ ounces carrier oil
```

Blend all the essential oils, then add them to a carrier oil of your choice. Store the mixtures in a dark-colored 2-ounce glass bottle with a spray lid. As a bonus, this blend is also soothing to bug bites. If you are bitten, swab a small amount onto the affected area for quick relief.

CANDLES

Citronella Insect Repellent Candle

....

If you are new to making candles with essential oils, purchase a candle-making kit from a craft store or online. Instead of using the chemical scents that come with the candle-making kit, use this insect-repelling aromatherapy blend. For best results, follow all the candle-making instructions exactly.

```
5 drops citronella essential oil
5 drops eucalyptus oil
```

Blend the essential oils. This recipe will scent 2 cups of soy wax flakes or the equivalent.

Rose Romance Candle

....

Perfect for the bedroom, this aromatherapy blend is designed to open the heart and awaken the senses.

```
6 drops sandalwood essential oil
2 drops rose otto essential oil
2 drops ylang-ylang essential oil
```

Blend the essential oils. This recipe will scent 2 cups of soy wax flakes or the equivalent.

Uplifting Citrus-Sage Candle

....

To bring positive energy into your home, burn a citrus-sage candle. Both the citrus and sage essential oils lift the spirits and promote feelings of well-being.

```
5 drops sweet orange essential oil
3 drops clary sage essential oil
2 drops lemon essential oil
```

Blend the essential oils. This recipe will scent 2 cups of soy wax flakes or the equivalent.

Cold Therapy Candle

If you are suffering from a cold, burning a candle made with essential oils can provide some relief. This fragrance uses peppermint and lavender essential oils, both of which are renowned for their usefulness in natural cold remedies.

```
7 drops lavender essential oil
3 drops peppermint essential oil
```

Blend the essential oils. This recipe will scent 2 cups of soy wax flakes or the equivalent.

Natural Holiday Candle

Enhance feelings of good cheer around the holidays with this delightful candle. Fir needle essential oil can help ease cold symptoms, making this a useful candle as well as a pleasant-smelling one.

```
8 drops fir needle essential oil
1 drop cinnamon essential oil
1 drop peppermint essential oil
```

Blend the essential oils. This recipe will scent 2 cups of soy wax flakes or the equivalent.

Meditative Mood Candle

....

If you enjoy meditating, use this candle to help bring on a meditative mood and enhance your meditation session. Both frankincense and helichrysum are known to promote enlightenment.

```
5 drops frankincense essential oil
5 drops helichrysum essential oil
```

Blend the essential oils. This recipe will scent 2 cups of soy wax flakes or the equivalent.

CLEANING SUPPLIES

Natural Window Cleaner

....

Instead of using chemical cleaners on windows, countertops, and other shiny surfaces, try this delightful and natural window cleaner. As a bonus, the lemon essential oil leaves an uplifting fragrance behind.

```
4 tablespoons white vinegar
12 drops lemon essential oil
Distilled water
```

Mix the vinegar and essential oil together in a clean 22-ounce spray bottle. Fill the bottle with distilled water. Shake well before each use.

Deodorizing Kitchen and Bathroom Cleaner

Rather than using harsh chemical cleaners, put the cleaning power and fragrance of this deodorizing kitchen and bathroom cleaner to work. Lavender, tea tree, and lemon essential oils are antibacterial, so your kitchen and bath will stay clean and sanitary.

```
5 drops lavender essential oil
5 drops lemon essential oil
5 drops tea tree essential oil
1/4 ounce liquid castile soap
18 ounces distilled water
```

Blend all the essential oils, and combine them with the castile soap. Use a funnel to pour the mixture into a 22-ounce spray bottle. Add the water and swirl gently to blend. Keep swirling until completely blended. Use to clean toilets and sinks.

Disinfecting Echinacea Cleaner

This recipe is a natural alternative to disinfecting cleaners that contain chemicals. The echinacea and lavender essential oils it contains help disinfect surfaces, killing bacteria and preventing the spread of viruses.

```
20 drops echinacea essential oil
20 drops lavender essential oil
8 ounces hydrogen peroxide
```

Blend the essential oils; add them to the hydrogen peroxide. Store in a glass bottle with a spray top, and shake vigorously before each use. To use, simply spray surfaces and allow the mixture to sit for about 15 seconds. Wipe dry with a clean cloth.

Nontoxic Bleach Alternative

....

For white laundry and sparkling clean surfaces throughout your home, give this nontoxic, non-irritating bleach alternative a try. The lemon essential oil leaves a lovely fragrance behind and helps impart a shine to solid surfaces.

1½ cups hydrogen peroxide
½ cup white vinegar
12 drops lemon essential oil
Water

Using a funnel, pour the hydrogen peroxide and vinegar into a clean 1-gallon jug. Add the essential oil, and swirl vigorously to blend. Fill the jug almost to the top with water. This is an excellent cleaner for toilets, sinks, and bathtubs. Add 1 cup to the laundry for softer, brighter clothing, and pre-treat stains by spraying a small amount onto clothing prior to laundering.

Natural Disinfecting Spray

....

This natural disinfecting spray is an excellent substitute for toxic chemicals. Both the tea tree and lemon essential oils in this blend have strong antibacterial capacities.

1½ cups distilled water
5 drops lemon essential oil
5 drops tea tree essential oil

Pour the distilled water into a clean spray bottle. Add the essential oils and shake well to blend. Spray on countertops and other surfaces, allow to sit for 15 seconds, and then wipe up with a paper towel or soft cloth. This spray is also great for disinfecting smelly garbage cans.

Gentle Scouring Solution

....

Use this gentle scouring solution in place of toxic commercial blends whenever stuck-on messes or even soapy bathtub rings are causing headaches for you. It will not scratch most surfaces; conduct a quick test before use if you are concerned that it may scratch. The grapefruit and lemon essential oils it contains disinfect while imparting a bright, pleasant fragrance.

$\frac{1}{2}$ cup baking soda
Liquid castile soap
10 drops grapefruit essential oil
10 drops lemon essential oil

Place the baking soda in a glass bowl. Add the soap, a small amount at a time, until a smooth paste forms. Add the essential oils and start scrubbing. This solution can be stored in an airtight glass jar; if it hardens, just add a small amount of water to reconstitute it.

Deodorizing Carpet Powder

....

This fragrant deodorizing carpet powder eliminates unpleasant carpet odors. The bergamot essential oil it contains leaves a fresh, uplifting scent behind and discourages bacteria.

2 cups baking soda
36 drops bergamot essential oil

Pour the baking soda into a glass bowl. Add the essential oil, a little at a time. Once blended, pour the mixtures into a glass jar or sugar shaker with a tight-fitting lid. Sprinkle it onto the carpet before vacuuming.

Lemon Furniture Polish

....

Keeping wood furniture looking good without resorting to toxic sprays is simple, thanks to this lemon furniture polish. The jojoba oil moisturizes wood, while the lemon essential oil imparts a fantastic shine and a wonderful fragrance.

```
1 teaspoon jojoba oil
20 drops lemon essential oil
6 tablespoons white vinegar
```

Blend the jojoba oil and essential oil; add the blended oils to the white vinegar in a 2-ounce glass bottle with a spray top. Shake vigorously before applying to furniture. Use a soft cloth to remove dust and polish wood surfaces.

PET PRODUCTS

Pet-Calming Aromatherapy Spray

....

If pets become nervous around strangers, while riding in the car, during thunderstorms, or at other times, use this calming aromatherapy spray to help reduce stress. Ylang-ylang essential oil has a wonderfully calming effect and is safe for dogs, cats, and horses.

```
8 drops ylang-ylang essential oil
4 drops distilled water
```

Blend the essential oil and water together in a glass spray bottle with a spray top. Lightly mist your pet's bedding and the air in areas where your pet spends time to promote a sense of calm.

Tick Repellent for Dogs

Ticks carry deadly diseases. Try this simple remedy if you dislike the idea of using chemical tick repellent on your dog; palo santo essential oil not only repels ticks but is good for aiding in their removal if they become attached.

```
10 drops palo santo essential oil
50 drops carrier oil
```

Blend the essential oil with a carrier oil of your choice in a 1-ounce spray bottle. Apply the mixtures to the dog's fur and rub gently. Use this solution every few days to keep ticks at bay. As a bonus, your dog will smell fantastic!

Lavender Flea Repellent for Dogs and Cats

If you're looking for a nontoxic alternative to commercial flea products, try this lavender flea repellent. As a bonus, the lavender will help any flea bites heal, and pets enjoy the calming fragrance of lavender.

```
20 drops lavender essential oil
Distilled water
```

Blend the essential oil and water in a 2-ounce spray bottle. Shake well before applying to pets. For skittish cats, apply the blend to your hands then gently wipe it onto the pet's fur. Keep away from eyes.

Keep Away Blend

....

If you don't want to choose between your furniture and your pets, try this fragrant blend. Neither rosemary essential oil nor peppermint essential oil is toxic to pets, but they dislike the fragrance.

```
10 drops rosemary essential oil
10 drops peppermint essential oil
```

Blend the essential oils. This mixture can be diffused to keep pets out of certain rooms, and it can be applied to furniture and other items to keep pets away. Add the oil mixture to a 2-ounce bottle, and fill almost to the top with distilled water to create a spray for sofas, chairs, and bedding you'd like to keep pet-free.

Pet-Safe Carpet Powder

....

If you enjoy having pets in your home but dislike pet hair, odor, and the occasional flea, give this pet-safe carpet powder a try. The lavender essential oil it contains is a natural flea repellant.

```
2 cups baking soda
36 drops lavender essential oil
```

Pour the baking soda into a glass bowl, add the essential oil, a little at a time. Once blended, pour the mixture into a glass jar or sugar shaker with a tight-fitting lid. Sprinkle onto the carpet before vacuuming.

Conclusion

You don't have to be an expert to begin enjoying the many benefits essential oils provide. If you're not sure where to begin, start with a few simple, inexpensive oils that have multiple uses. You'll find many ways to use lemon, lavender, and peppermint essential oils for everything from headaches to body detoxification.

When you feel comfortable with those oils, add a few more to your collection. Some of the most useful include orange, tea tree, and rosemary essential oils. By adding these, you'll broaden your ability to use essential oils in a variety of ways.

Remember, a small amount of essential oil is all it takes to make a difference. When preparing the recipes and aromatherapy blends recommended in this book, follow the instructions for combining and using the oils. Using more than recommended can have an adverse effect.

Finally, remember that not all essential oils are equally effective. The market is flooded with many cheap substitutes that are at best ineffective, and at worst harmful. Select a reputable source for essential oils and you'll ensure that the natural remedies you try will be as effective and safe as possible.

Armed with a handful of powerful essential oils and the knowledge this book contains, you can begin living a healthier and more sustainable lifestyle. Best of all, each of the recipes contained within these pages is a real pleasure to use, so you just might find that life is more enjoyable when you make the decision to begin replacing commercial products with natural ones you can make at home.

Glossary

adaptogen: a substance that promotes a healing reaction within the body

analgesic: any substance that relieves pain by acting on the nervous system

anesthetic: a substance that eases pain while simultaneously promoting relaxation

antibacterial: a substance that inhibits bacterial growth

anti-catarrhal: a substance that helps to ease inflammation associated with upper respiratory infections, and is often used in combination with expectorants and/or mucolytic agents

anticonvulsant: a substance that may prevent or decrease convulsions

antiemetic: a substance that aids in treating nausea and vomiting

antifungal: a substance that inhibits fungal growth

anti-infectious: a substance that has the potential to eliminate both viruses and bacteria

anti-inflammatory: a substance or treatment that reduces inflammation

antimicrobial: a substance that inhibits microbial growtha

antineuritic: a substance that acts to inhibit inflammation of the nerves

antirheumatic: a substance that relieves or prevents rheumatism

antiseptic: a substance that inhibits the growth of microorganisms

antispasmodic: a substance that relieves or prevents spasms, particularly smooth-muscle spasms

antitumoral: a substance that counteracts or prevents the formation of tumors

antitussive: a substance that is used to suppress coughing

antiviral: a substance that helps prevent the spread of viruses

aromatherapy: a form of alternative medicine in which essential oils are used to positively influence a person's mind, bodily health, mood, or cognitive function

astringent: a compound that shrinks bodily tissues

Ayurveda: traditional Indian medical science dating to 3000 BCE and still in use today

balsamic: an essential oil that soothes scratchy or sore throats

carminative: a substance that prevents or inhibits the formation of intestinal gas

cephalic: a substance that aids in promoting good digestion

cicatrizant: a substance that promotes healing through scar tissue formation

cordial: suitable for use in a medicinal beverage

demulcent: a substance that soothes irritated mucus membranes

depurative: a substance that has both purifying and detoxifying properties

diaphoretic: a substance that promotes sweating

diffusion: using a diffuser or spray bottle to blend essential oils with a small amount of water for dispersal through the air

direct inhalation: inhaling essential oils directly into the nostrils rather than diffusing them

diuretic: a substance that promotes urine production

emmenagogue: a substance that stimulates blood flow, particularly in the uterine region

enfleurage: an old-fashioned method of extracting essential oils that is still in use on a limited basis

expectorant: a substance that promotes or facilitates the expulsion of mucus or phlegm

expression: a method of extracting essential oils, usually citrus

febrifuge: a substance that reduces fevers

grading: a method of ascertaining which essential oils are suitable for certain purposes

hepatic: a substance that assists in liver detoxification

hypercritical carbon dioxide extraction: a method of producing high-quality essential oils

hypertensive: a substance that can cause an increase in blood pressure

hypotensive: a substance that can cause a decrease in blood pressure

inflammation: part of the body's natural immune response normally characterized by swelling, redness, or pain

mucolytic: a substance that may loosen mucus and aid in clearing airways

neat: undiluted

nervine: a substance that calms the nerves; can refer to a sedative

patch test: a test to confirm whether one is sensitive to an essential oil or not; simply dab a small amount of essential oil or diluted essential oil onto the skin and wait twenty-four hours to see whether sensitivity occurs

pectoral: a substance that relieves discomfort of the respiratory tract or chest

phototoxin: a substance that causes extra sensitivity to sunlight and UV light

purity: pure essential oils that have not been adulterated or diluted

restorative: a substance that restores feelings of health, well-being, or both

rubefacient: a substance that produces skin redness

solvent: chemical solution of extracting essential oils

steam distillation: a popular method of extracting essential oils

stomachic: a substance that improves stomach function or increases appetite

styptic: a substance capable of contracting tissues or blood vessels to control light bleeding

sudorific: a substance that causes sweating

tonic: a substance that invigorates the body or promotes health

topical application: the act of applying a substance to the skin

vasodilator: a substance which causes widening of the blood vessels

vermifuge: a substance capable of purging intestinal parasites from the body

viscosity: thickness

volatile oils: another term for essential oils

vulnerary: a substance that is useful in healing wounds

Recommended Reading

Heidi Corley Barto, *The Natural Soap Chef: Making Luxurious Delights from Cucumber Melon and Almond Cookie to Chai Tea and Espresso Forte* (Ulysses Press, 2012)

If you love the idea of making soaps for your own consumption or to present as gifts, you will enjoy *The Natural Soap Chef.* This book contains step-by-step instructions for making luxurious soaps, plus beautiful photographs to help enhance your understanding of the process.

Kristen Leigh Bell, *Holistic Aromatherapy for Animals: A Comprehensive Guide to the Use of Essential Oils and Hydrosols with Animals* (Findhorn Press, 2002)

An outstanding resource for anyone who enjoys companion animals, *Holistic Aromatherapy for Animals* is an excellent guide to maintaining animal health the natural way. It contains an impressive amount of aromatherapy information as well as numerous treatments for common illnesses.

Jennie Harding, *The Essential Oils Handbook: All the Oils You Will Ever Need for Health, Vitality, and Well-Being* (Duncan Baird, 2008)

The Essential Oils Handbook provides a comprehensive directory of one hundred essential oils and a thorough discussion of each essential oil presented. Beautiful photographs make this book a pleasure to read.

Kathi Keville and Mindy Green, *Aromatherapy: A Complete Guide to the Healing Art*, 2nd edition (Crossing Press, 2009)

This book details a variety of methods for using essential oils in health and beauty as well as for total well-being. It is suitable for beginners as well as for those with a background in aromatherapy, and it contains more than ninety formulas for essential oils.

Julia Lawless, *The Illustrated Encyclopedia of Essential Oils: The Complete Guide to the Use of Oils in Aromatherapy and Herbalism,* 2nd edition (Element Books Ltd., 1995)

This well-organized encyclopedia provides many uses for plants and essential oils. It is regarded as one of the best-respected reference books on the topic of aromatherapy.

Carol Schiller and David Schiller, *500 Formulas for Aromatherapy: Mixing Essential Oils for Every Use* (Sterling, 1994)

An excellent recipe book that contains hundreds of blends, this comprehensive guide to using essential oils is well organized and will prove useful to anyone hoping to reduce reliance on commercially prepared products. Hair care, body care, aromatherapy blends, and household solutions are all well represented.

Kurt Schnaubelt, *Advanced Aromatherapy: The Science of Essential Oil Therapy* (Healing Arts Press, 1998)

Advanced Aromatherapy provides clear, logical explanations about how essential oils work. In addition, this book provides a scientific basis for the efficacy of essential oils, with clear references to how they work on the body's cellular structure and how they affect microbes.

Kurt Schnaubelt, *The Healing Intelligence of Essential Oils: The Science of Advanced Aromatherapy* (Healing Arts Press, 2011)

This well-written book enhances biological understanding of how essential oils treat diseases and improve immunity. Not for the uninitiated, it is excellent for anyone who is ready to take aromatherapy to the next level.

Valerie Ann Worwood, *Aromatherapy for the Healthy Child: More Than 300 Natural, Nontoxic, and Fragrant Essential Oil Blends* (New World Library, 2000)

Aromatherapy for the Healthy Child is an outstanding reference for parents who hope to raise happy, healthy children the natural way. With hundreds of aromatherapy treatments for a wide range of conditions, this book is designed for parents of children ranging in age from newborn to teen.

Valerie Ann Worwood, *The Complete Book of Essential Oils and Aromatherapy: Over 600 Natural, Nontoxic, and Fragrant Recipes to Create Health, Beauty, and a Safe Home Environment* (New World Library, 1991)

This is an excellent resource for anyone with an interest in expanding their knowledge about essential oils and aromatherapy. It contains easy-to-follow recipes for treating many common conditions.

Resources

AUTHENTIC ESSENTIAL OIL RETAILERS

Aura Cacia

Founded in 1981, Aura Cacia provides authentic essential oils, including therapeutic-quality oils and premium essential oil blends, as well as many organic options. All products contain 100 percent pure essential oils to ensure users receive appropriate aromatherapy benefits. *www.auracacia.com*

Aura Cacia
5398 31st Avenue
Urbana, IA 52345
1-800-437-3301

dōTERRA Essential Oils

dōTERRA carries only certified pure therapeutic-grade essential oils without fillers or artificial ingredients. Founded in 2008, dōTERRA now offers products through independent consultants who maintain personal online shopping sites and who offer local distribution in some areas. Single oils, essential oil blends, accessories, and other products are available. *www.doterra.com*

dōTERRA International, LLC
370 West Center
Orem, UT 84057
1-801-615-7200

Mountain Rose Herbs

Mountain Rose Herbs has been producing whole herbs and essential oils since 1987. All products are 100 percent pure and 100 percent authentic. Mountain Rose Herbs is a certified organic processor through Oregon Tilth, which is fully accredited with the USDA National Organic Program. Bulk ingredients are available, as are containers and other items designed for working with and storing essential oils and blends.
www.mountainroseherbs.com

Mountain Rose Herbs
PO Box 50220
Eugene, OR 97405
1-800-879-3337

NOW Foods

NOW Foods provides a wide range of pure essential oils of the highest quality available. Many of these products are sold in natural food stores and in other retail locations. NOW is an excellent source for many of the most popular essential oils and carrier oils; all oils are laboratory tested and are guaranteed to be 100 percent pure.
www.nowfoods.com

NOW Foods
244 Knollwood Drive, Suite 300
Bloomingdale, IL 60108
1-888-669-3663

Young Living Essential Oils

Young Living carries a vast range of essential oils and essential oil blends as well as carrier oils, diffusers, and much more. All the essential oils Young Living carries are 100 percent pure and authentic. These products are available online or from an independent distributor in your area.
www.youngliving.com

Young Living Essential Oils
Thanksgiving Point Business Park
3125 Executive Parkway
Lehi, UT 84043
1-800-371-3515

EDUCATION AND LEARNING

American College of Healthcare Science

Founded in New Zealand in 1978, American College of Healthcare Science (ACHS) opened its United States campus in 1989. ACHS offers online holistic health education and is accredited by the Distance Education and Training Council. ACHS offers certificate, diploma, undergraduate, and graduate degree programs.
www.achs.edu

American College of Healthcare Science
5940 SW Hood Avenue
Portland, OR 97239
1-800-487-8839

California School of Herbal Studies

Offering hands-on studies in herbalism, herbal pharmacy, herbal skin formulation, and much more, the California School of Herbal Studies is located on eighty acres in Sonoma County, California. Classes vary by season, so check the school's website for current information.
www.cshs.com

California School of Herbal Studies
PO Box 39
Forestville, CA 95436
1-707-887-7457

East West School of Planetary Herbology

The East West School of Planetary Herbology offers a unique approach to herbal medicine, integrating diagnostic tools and plants from all over the world. Webinars and correspondence courses are available, covering a wide range of topics related to herbalism and holistic health.
www.planetherbs.com

East West School of Planetary Herbology
PO Box 275
Ben Lomond, CA 95005
1-800-717-5010

Florida School of Holistic Living

Founded in 1999, the Florida School of Holistic Living offers classes in herbalism as well as courses covering a wide range of holistic living topics, from beekeeping to permaculture. Distance learning programs are available. Check the school's website for current offerings.
www.holisticlivingschool.org

Florida School of Holistic Living
1109 East Concord Street
Orlando, FL 32803
1-407-595-3731

Southwest Institute of Healing Arts

Southwest Institute of Healing Arts is a nationally accredited private college as well as a community healing center for holistic healthcare careers and continuing education. Single courses, certificate programs, and degrees are available in fields such as Western herbalism, bodywork, massage therapy, and more.
www.swiha.edu

Southwest Institute of Healing Arts
1100 East Apache Boulevard
Tempe, AZ 85281
1-888-504-9106

References

Chevallier, Andrew. *Encyclopedia of Herbal Medicine: The Definitive Home Reference Guide to 550 Key Herbs with All Their Uses as Remedies for Common Ailments,* 2nd rev. ed. New York, NY: DK Publishing Inc, 2000.

Edwards, Victoria H. *The Aromatherapy Companion: Medicinal Uses, Ayurvedic Healing, Body-Care Blends, Perfumes and Scents, Emotional Health and Well-Being.* North Adams, MA: Storey Publishing, 1999.

Foster, Steven, and James A. Duke. *A Field Guide to Medicinal Plants and Herbs of Eastern and Central North America,* 2nd rev. ed. New York, NY: Houghton Mifflin Company, 2000.

Gladstar, Rosemary. *Rosemary Gladstar's Medicinal Herbs: A Beginner's Guide.* North Adams, MA: Storey Publishing, 2012.

Keville, Kathi, and Mindy Green. *Aromatherapy: A Complete Guide to the Healing Art,* 2nd ed. New York, NY: Crossing Press, 2009.

Worwood, Valerie Ann. *The Complete Book of Essential Oils and Aromatherapy: Over 600 Natural, Nontoxic, and Fragrant Recipes to Create Health, Beauty, and a Safe Home Environment.* Novato, CA: New World Library, 1991.

Worwood, Valerie Ann. *The Fragrant Mind: Aromatherapy for Personality, Mind, Mood and Emotion.* Novato, CA: New World Library, 1996.

Index

CPSIA information can be obtained
at www.ICGtesting.com
Printed in the USA
BVHW070145031118
531993BV00001B/1/P